ENCYCLOPAEDIA OF AIDS AND SEXUAL BEHAVIOUR

ENCYCLOPAEDIA OF AIDS AND SEXUAL BEHAVIOUR

VOL. 3

Edited by

B.K. Sinha

ANMOL PUBLICATIONS PVT. LTD.
NEW DELHI-110 002 (INDIA)

ANMOL PUBLICATIONS PVT. LTD.
4374/4B, Ansari Road, Daryaganj
New Delhi - 110 002

Encyclopaedia of AIDS and Sexual Behaviour

First Edition, 1999
ISBN 81-261-0330-2 (Set)

PRINTED IN INDIA

Published by J.L. Kumar for Anmol Publications Pvt. Ltd., New Delhi and Printed at Mehra Offset Press, Delhi.

S

sack coitus an unusual technique in which one partner has placed himself or herself in a rubber or other sack.

secret area a segment of the spinal cord in the lower back where nerve centres that control penile erection and ejaculation are located. Because sexual stimulation is controlled in part by the brain, men who have suffered spinal injuries are frequently able to achieve partial or complete erections, and many are able to have successful intercourse.

sacred prostitution an early religious custom in which prostitutes dedicated themselves to the service of fertility gods or goddesses. These women performed sexual acts with priests or, in some instances, with worshippers, inside the temple. The practice has been traced as far back as the 5th century B C and was at one time common in Babylonia, Arabia, Greece, India, and West Africa. It has been conjectured that prostitution itself may have started as a sacred rite and only later became secularized. Also called temple prostitution.

sacred triangle the triangular mound above the vulva; the mons veneris or mons pubis.

sacrum the bones of the sacral vertebrae, which in adult life are a fused mass of separate vertebrae. The sacrum forms a smooth concave surface below the small of the back and represents the back of the pelvis.

sadism a psychosexual disorder, or paraphilia, in which sexual excitement is obtained by inflicting pain on the sexual partner. Sadistic acts may consist of physical cruelty, such as flogging or bondage, or mental cruelty, as in humiliating the partner. The suffering may be inflicted on either a consenting or a nonconsenting person, and may range from mild injury to raping, torturing, or even killing the victim.

sadomasochism a complementary relationship in which one person derives pleasure and usually sexual gratification from inflicting pain while the other becomes sexually aroused by experiencing that pain.

safe a slang term for condom.

safe period a popular term for the days of the menstrual cycle when conception is lent likely to result from intercourse without use of a contraceptive device.

saint's delight a colloquial term for vagina.

saliromania a compulsive need to obtain sexual gratification through preoccupation with filth, ugliness, or deformity. Examples are soiling one's partner or oneself, watching mud-wrestling bouts between women, viewing grotesquely deformed persons at fairs, getting a 'kick' out of anal or urinary odours, or, more mildly, using obscene, 'dirty' words during sexual foreplay. The most extreme form of this paraphilia is coprophagia.

Many Freudians trace saliromania to an unsatisfied urge to play with faeces at about 2 years of age.

salpingectomy the surgical removal of a uterine, or fallopian, tube. An incision into a fallopian tube is a salpingotomy. A salpingectomy accompanied by surgical removal of an ovary is termed a salpingo-oophorectomy.

selpingitis an inflammation of the fallopian tubes. The condition may be marked by pain on one or both sides, infrequent episodes of nausea, excessive menstrual flow, and a fever that may rise to 104°F. Causes may include hypersensitivity to an IUD, or an infection, such as gonorrhoea or tuberculosis. Salpingitis from gonorrhoea often is associated with an abnormal discharge or painful or difficult urination, particularly just before the start of a menstrual period.

salpingitis isthmica nodosa a disorder of the fallopian tubes marked by the development of nodules and abnormally thickened walls in the portion of the tube that is attached to the uterus.

salpingotomy a surgical procedure in which an incision is made into a fallopian tube.

saltpetre a common name for potassium nitrate, a substance that has been used as a diuretic and to induce sweating. It is an ancient medication, included in prescriptions on Sumerian tablets of 4,000 years ago, but potentially harmful as a precursor of nitrosamine carcinogens, as a destroyer of red blood cells, and as a lethal poison, despite its legendary application as an anaphrodisiac.

some-sex sex play the tendency of children to adopt, in play with other children of the opposite sex, rolls identified with older members of their own sex. A boy and girl may agree to 'play house,' a game in which the boy plays the father role and the girl the role of the mother. The game may include coital play in which the boy ties on top of the girl in imitation of scenes from their own home or in films or television.

Samoans inhabitants of a group of islands in Western Polynesia. Monogamy is the rule except for chiefs, who usually have several wives. Other practices include sex hospitality: adolescent homosexuality, which is regarded as an innocent form of play; decorating the bodies with tattoos, a custom that is on the decline today; and night-crawling by unpopular and desperate young men-a practice that Margaret Mead called surreptitious rape', and which led to outright shunning by other girls if they were caught.

Sanger, Margaret an American leader of the birth-control movement. Building on wide experience as an obstetrical nurse for underprivileged families and single mothers. Sanger decided that the high infant-and-adult-mortality rates, especially found in self-induced abortions, could only be combatted by liberating women from unwanted pregnancies. Accordingly, and in defiance of the Comstock Act, she began publicizing contraceptive methods in a magazine she founded in 1914, the Woman Rebel; she published a widely read pamphlet, Family Limitation, and in 1921 founded the American Birth Control League. In 1927 she organized the first World Population Conference in Geneva, and in 1936 was instrumental in modification of the Comstock Act to permit doctors to prescribe contraceptives. Her work then spread to over-populated countries, and in 1953 she was elected first president of the International Planned Parenthood Federation.

sanitary towel a disposable pad made of cellulose or cotton designed to absorb the menstrual flow when held in place along the opening of the vagina by panties, a belt or adhesive backing that sticks to the panties.

sapphism an alternative for Iesbianism based on the fact that the Greek poetess Sappho lived on the island of Lesbos and wrote lyrical poems about love and sex, generally assumed to be between women.

sarcoma botyroides a type of vaginal cancer that may appear as grapelike clusters of tissue. Untreated, the growth may eventually protrude from the opening of the vagina. It also is likely to be accompanied by bleeding.

sarcoma of the prostate a rare form of prostatic tumour that may affect men at any age but occurs most often in infants and small boys. In infant boys, the treatment usually is surgical removal of the prostate, seminal vesicles, and urinary bladder. The urinary system is rebuilt so that urine is diverted through the intestinal tract.

Sarcoptes scabiel a mite that burrows between the layers of skin to deposit eggs, resulting in a skin rash that itches and may produce pimples and pustules. The condition, called scabies, can be transmitted by sexual contact in the same manner as crab lice.

sard the oldest English term for having sexual intercourse, from around 950 A.D.

sathon in ancient Greece, a boy loved by an older man.

satiation a state of complete satisfaction or gratification of sexual or other drives, such as hunger or thirst.

sattvic foods foods that, according to practitioners of yoga, stimulate the creative and erotic senses. They include milk, butter, honey, nuts, grains, most fruits, and the vegetables that grow above ground. Sattvic foods are related to the sweet taste, and reportedly result in a sweet, nonirritating semen that is best for a healthy offspring.

satyriasis a male psychosexual disorder characterized by an obsessive, insatiable desire for sexual gratification. The condition is not the result of being physically 'oversexed,' but stems from unconscious emotional needs, such as the need for reassurance of potency, an attempt to deny homosexual tendencies, a means of alleviating anxiety, or a need to compensate for failures or inadequacies in other areas of life. The term itself is derived from the satyrs of Greek mythology, who were alleged to be part human and part animal, and to have an unlimited sex drive.

saucer edge medical Jargon for the breasts of women with adenosis, a lymph-gland disorder. The breasts tend to be small, dense, and filled with tiny nodules which give them the feel of the edge of a saucer when palpated.

sauna club often a euphemism for massage parlour.

scarification the process of producing a scar, or cicatrix, as in making superficial cuts in the surface of the skin. Scarification is found among many African societies, where it is used as a means of beautifying the skin and making the individual more sexually desirable.

scarlet woman an obsolete euphemism for loose woman.

scatography the practice of writing any kind of material, including graffiti, relating to eliminative functions, as a means of expressing or arousing sexual interest.

scatology the study of or interest in excrement, filth, and obscenity. Scatological language is sometimes used as a stimulant during sexual encounters, especially those involving anal eroticism. Also called *scatologia.*

scatophobia another term for penis. The term is also used figuratively, referring to someone who is considered to be stupid or silly.

Schrenck-Natzing, Albert von a Viennese psychiatrist who helped pave the way for acceptance of Freud's theories, but was particularly noted for his attempts to modify the sexual orientation of homosexuals through hypnotic suggestion and visits to brothels, where they might be reconditioned to heterosexual relationships.

scirrhus a form of cancer of the prostate that is identified by its hardness when palpated through the rectum by an examining doctor. A scirrhus cancer may also occur in the breast.

sclerosing lymphangitis of the penis an inflammation of the lymphatic vessels of the shaft of the penis. The condition is characterized by an enlargement and hardening of the lymph vessels resulting in a cordlike thickening of the lymph ducts near the corona glandis.

Scold's bridal an alternative term for brank, a gag used for taming shrews and, more recently, for bondage games.

scopophilia a sexual variance in which gratification is achieved by viewing the sexual activities or sexual organs of others. Freud distinguished between an active and a passive form of scopophilia—that is, pleasure in looking and pleasure in being looked at. If this deviation is a persistent or exclusive source of gratification, it is essentially equivalent to voyeurism. Also called scoptophilia; scotophilia.

scopophobla a morbid fear of being looked at. It is an extreme form of shyness usually occurring in adolescence and resulting from sexual self-consciousness.

scoptolagnia sexual excitement produced by looking at nude persons or exposed genitalia.

scoptophilia an alternative term for scopophilia.

score a slang term meaning to achieve sexual success, particularly in persuading a woman to have sex with one-thus a man might be asked 'Did you score last night?'

scoptophilia an alternative term for scopophilia.

scrape an Australian slang term meaning to copulate.

screw a slang term used either as a verb, meaning to copulate, or as a noun, meaning sexual intercourse or partner in interlockers. In addition it is used metaphorically in phrases like screw you!, an expletive, and screw up, meaning to botch.

scrotal angioma a type of tumour of the scrotum marked by wartlike growths associated with a disorder involving dilated blood vessels of the skin.

scrotal erysipelas an infection of the scrotal skin and subcutaneous tissues caused, as in most other types of erysipelas, by a streptococcal organism. It results from wounds and abscesses, and as secondary disorders is associated with chancroid or other diseases, such as lymphatic infections. The scrotum becomes smooth, swollen, and warm, with small blisters on the surface.

scrotal hypospedia a congenital malformation in which the outlet of the male urethra is between the testicles. The scrotum in such cases is usually associated with imperfectly descended testes.

scrotal pouch the pocket of membrane that precedes the descent of the testes into the scrotum during the seventh month of gestation. The membranous pouch leaves the abdominal cavity and migrates into the primitive skin sac that will become the scrotum, to serve as one of the inner layers of the scrotum.

scrotal temperature the temperature of the scrotum, which normally is slightly lower than body temperature. The lower temperature is necessary for the production of viable spermatozoa. The scrotum is quite temperature-sensitive, tending to move farther away from the body in a warm environment such as a hot bath but moving closer to the body in cold temperatures.

scrotal xanthomata a type of eruptive xanthomata, or skin lesions, that may appear on the surface of the scrotum and other genital and perineal areas in cases of hypertriglyceridaemia, a condition of extremely excessive blood fats. The lesions resemble the skin sores associated with chicken pox.

scrotitis an inflammation of the scrotum. The causes may include a number of infections, such as mumps, gonorrhoea, typhoid fever, scarlet fever, influenza, syphilis, leprosy, tuberculosis, or brucellosis. Other possible causes include injury, a hernia with a segment of the intestine incarcerated in the scrotum, undescended testicle with referred pain, a tumour, gout, rheumatic fever, hydrocele, or torsion of the spermatic cord. The scrotum also could be the site of referred pain from appendicitis or a kidney stone. The scrotal pain may be mild or excruciating.

scrotopexy a surgical procedure in which a portion of the scrotum is removed to correct a defect. The operation is usually combined with scrotoplasty, or the use of plastic surgery to refashion the scrotum.

scrotum a pouch of skin and related supportive tissues containing the male testis, epididymides, and portions of the spermatic cord. It is located near the bulb of the penis and in the pubic area of the perineum. The scrotum is divided by a wall of tissue, and because the left spermatic cord is longer, the left side is normally lower than the right side. The scrotum is generally translucent, meaning a beam of light from one side will illuminate the scrotal contents in a darkened room.

scrubber a British derogatory slang term for a prostitute, or more generally for any woman with accommodating sexual morals.

seafood a male homosexual slang term for a homosexual sailor.

seasonal sex a term referring to the idea that human sexual activity, like mating in 90 percent of the animal kingdom, is a seasonal function. There is, however, little if any evidence for a biologically based human 'rutting season,' but there are variations caused by other factors. Among the

Eskimos more intercourse takes place during long winter nights than during the summer, and among Westerners, as a whole, more children are conceived in the summer when holidays occur.

seated sex sexual intercourse with one or both partners in a sitting position. Usually the man sits in a chair or on the edge of a bed, and the woman lowers herself on him; his pelvic movements are restricted, but his hands are free. The woman usually faces the man but may have her back to him; she may also sit on him as he lies on his back.

sebaceous cyst a sebum, gland cyst, similar to an acne swelling, that can develop in the labia majora or minora. The labia are well supplied with the sebaceous oil glands. If one or more become blocked by skin-cell debris, a tender, painful furuncle will develop at the site. Untreated, a sebaceous cyst of the labia can grow to the size of a walnut.

secondarism the seeking of sexual arousal through relations with a person who has just participated in a sex act.

secondary amenorrhoea a cessation of menses after they have become established. The cause may be an illness, change of environment, or surgical removal of the ovaries or uterus before menopause.

secondary erectile dysfunction a form of impotence in which a man is not able to produce or maintain an erection to perform intercourse, although he was previously able to produce a satisfactory erection. A major causal factor is psychological stress or conflict.

secondary hypogonadism a condition of male sexual

dysfunction that is related to a malfunction of brain-regulated testosterone production, as distinguished from a hormonal disorder caused by a defect in the testes.

secondary Impotence a condition in which a male has been able to achieve a normal erection and ejaculation in intercourse but is not able to repeat the performance. Technically, secondary impotence can occur after the first act of coitus, and nearly all men eventually encounter a time when they cannot repeat a sexual activity they may have performed thousands of times without failure. As a rule of thumb, secondary impotence is considered a problem only when a man fails to achieve an erection in 25 percent of attempts.

secondary oocyte a female gamete produced by meiotic division of a primary oocyte. The primary oocyte contains the diploid number of chromosomes and in dividing produces the secondary oocyte and one polar body, each with 23, or half the diploid number. The secondary ooctye undergoes mitosis to produce a mature ovum and a second polar body, each with the haploid number of chromosomes.

secondary orgasmic dysfunction a condition in which a woman or man has managed to achieve orgasm at least once, whether by coitus, masturbation or some other form of stimulation, but can no longer do so. Also called situational orgasmic dysfunction.

secondary sex characteristics physical characteristics other than the external sex organs that distinguish between male and female: texture of facial, body, and underarm hair; voice quality; size of the breasts and nipples; pattern of pubic hair; and body contours.

secondary testicular failure a male gonadal deficiency that results from failure of the pituitary gland to secrete gonadotropic hormones. Because the testes fail to receive the stimulating hormones, they remain in an infantile state. Secondary hypogonadism, or secondary testicular failure, accounts for more than three fourths of males afflicted with hypogonadism.

secondary wives in a polygynous society, women who serve as additional wives beyond the original or primary wife. These wives, or concubines, are recognized as sexual partners but not as managers of the household or even as mothers of the children, even though they may actually be the mothers.

second-stage orgasm the phase of ejaculation of semen by the male after the prostate, seminal vesicles, and ductus deferens have released their semen components into the dilated urethral bulb. Contractions of the muscles at the base of the penis and peristaltic action of the genital ducts combine to expel the semen forcefully from the urethral meatus during this phase of orgasm.

second testicular hormone a term applied to a speculative source of oestrogens found in the urine of men. Because male oestrogen occurs only in males with functionally active Leydig cells, it has been assumed that the cells produce a testicular hormone in addition to testosterone and that it is a form of oestrogen.

secret service a slang term for the work of a prostitute whose sexual services are clandestine, known only to her regular clients, but otherwise unknown even among her close acquaintances.

secret vice an older euphemism for masturbation.

seduction the enticing or inducing of a female into sexual intercourse without the use of force-for example, by promising marriage or by bribery. Seduction is considered a criminal act in some countries, usually when it involves an unmarried girl or woman.

seductive behaviour a form of unconscious incestuous behaviour, according to many psychotherapists, in which parental attitudes towards a child may be seductive. The parental behaviour may never culminate in overt incest, but it may condition the child to accept the role playing because of the implicit approval of the parents. The child may have little or no guilt until later in life when he or she learns from others that incest is forbidden.

segmentation the process of mitotic division of the zygote, or fertilized ovum, into 2, then 4, 8, 16, and soon daughter cells. The process, however, follows a pattern of cleavage planes whereby the second division, from 2 to 4 cells, occurs at right angles to the first phase of division. The third division occurs in a third plane, and so on, until the mass of small cells, called a morula, is ready for implantation into the wall of the uterus.

selective gonadotropic failure a condition caused by mild anterior-pituitary -gland insufficiency in the male and characterized by a penis, scrotum, and prostate that fail to grow to mature sizes. The body type of the individual is eunuchoid, with arms and leg, of abnormal proportions.

self-abuse an archaic, moralistic term for masturbation based on the antiquated notion that it is injurious or sinful.

self-castration another term for self-emasculation.

self-control the ability to exert restraint over ones impulses, especially to inhibit the sex urge, or delay orgasm until the partner is 'ready.'

self-emasculation a form of self-mutilation in which an individual castrates himself, usually as a religious or ascetic practice. Self-emasculation is' extremely rare today although it is occasionally found among psychotic patients who are suffering from a delusion of guilt. In the past there have been many cases in ancient Egypt, among the priests of Atzis in Greece, among medicine men in Asia and North America, among certain dervish sects, and in the Skoptsy sect of 18th-century Russia.

self-induced abortion abortion deliberately brought on by the pregnant woman, for example, by removing the embryo or foetus through the use of an instrument such as a corkscrew. Such methods are extremely dangerous and may result in serious illness or even death from blood poisoning.

self-mutilation a self-destructive act in which the individual severely injures or disfigures himself or herself as a form of expiation for real or fancied misdeeds, religious excess, or an extreme form of masochism. Examples are repetitive wrist cutting, burning the skin with a cigarette or flame, self-castration, or scarification.

self-pleasuring a recently adopted term for masturbation, or manipulation of the sex organs or other body areas for pleasure and for release of sexual tension.

self-pollution an obsolete term for masturbation.

self-stimulation a synonyrn for masturbation,

manipulation of the ex organs for the purpose of sexual excitement and gratification.

semen the fluid containing spermatozoa that is ejaculated by the male during intercourse. The fluid is produced by the prostate gland and seminal vesicles and contains substances that tend to increase the survivability of the spermatozoa in the female reproductive tract, such as an alkaline substance to neutralize the acidity of the vagina.

semen analysis laboratory examination of a sample of semen obtained in a wide-mouthed glass bottle after masturbation or coitus reservatus has been performed to produce an ejaculate. The patient abstains from sexual activity for 3 to 5 days before producing the semen sample. The semen is never collected in a rubber container because rubber is usually impregnated with chemicals that destroy spermtozoa. A sample of 3 to 5 millilitres should contain 100 to 120 million spermatozoa, of which 80 to 85 percent should be highly motile. And at least 80 percent of the spermatozoa should be normal in appearance. When fewer than 40 percent of the spermatozoa are actively motile and more than 20 percent are of abnormal shapes and sizes, the risk of subnormal fertility can often be explained. Abnormal spermatozoa may include microsperm, megalosperm, aplastic head, double head, double tail, and other forms. Spermatozoa of a normal healthy male usually contain a few abnormally shaped spermatozoa.

semen content a term usually referring to the total content of semen. The question of semen content arises especially among persons who regularly swallow semen, as in fellatio, and who are concerned about calorie intake and nutritional substances. The average ejaculate of about 4 cubic centimetres. weighing about 4 grams, contains less than 35 calories, mainly in proteins and fats, In all, semen contains tiny amounts of over 30 substances, none of which is harmful-including ammonia, ascorbic acid, blood-group antigens, calcium, chlorine, cholesterol, choline, citric acid, creatine, deoxyribonucleic acid (DNA), fructose, glutathione, hyaluronidase, inositol, lactic acid, magnesium, nitrogen, phosphorus, potass˘ium, purine, pyrimidine, pyruvic acid sodium, sorbitol, spermidine, spermine, urea uric acid, vitamin B12, zinc... For analysis of sperm.

semen myths fictitious beliefs and superstitions concerning semen, for example, the Hindu belief that the semen is the basis of health, strength, and long life, and should be conserved through periodic abstinence and through avoiding masturbation and nocturnal emissions as far as possible. Somewhat similarly, the early Chinese held that ejaculation diminished the yang, or male, element and therefore reduces the man's strength and may even shorten his life. Various methods were therefore used to retain as much semen as possible even during intercourse. A third example is the belief among the Etoro, in Oceania, that boys have no semen at birth but acquire enough semen for sexual activity through oral insemination by older men.

semen retention in early Taoist and Tantric treatises, the use of various techniques to regulate the emission of semen so that a Portion of it will 'ascend and nourish the brain'. Some Taoist masters recommend that ideally semen should be released only two or three times in ten sessions, and that certain lovemaking postures such as sitting, squatting, and having the man lie flat on his back, are especially effective in helping to control the semen, and in directing sexual energy upwards to the brain.

semenuria the presence of semen in the urine. The condition may result from semen reflux, or retrograde ejaculation, in which semen is forced into the urinary bladder as a result of effects of prostate surgery or a urethral defect, such as a stricture.

seminal cyst a cyst caused by retention of the sperm in the testis or epididymis.

seminal discharge the discharge of semen, during intercourse, masturbation, or nocturnal emission.

seminal duct an alternative name for the ductus deferens or vas deferens.

seminal vesicles a pair of membranous pouches embedded in the prostate gland and u iited with the ductus deferens at the ejaculatory ducts. The vesicles secrete a fluid that is combined at the ejaculatory ducts with the spermatozoa from the ductus deferens and added to the akaline secretions of the prostate gland. The seminal vesicles do not store spermatozoa as was previously believed. Each vesicle is actually a blind tube that coils upon itself so that its internal length is actually several times that of its external size of approximately 3 inches.

semination the deposition of semen in the vagina or uterus, either during intercourse or by artificial insemination.

seminiterous tubules the straight or convoluted tubes in the lobes of the testes. A testis is estimated to contain more than 800 of the tubules each of which may be 30 inches in length. In the walls of the convoluted tubules are spermatozoa in various stages of development and maturation.

seminoma a common type of testicular tumour with a cellular pattern that resembles the germinal cells in the seminferous tubules. Most of the tumours that develop in undescended testicles are seminomas.

senile ovary the ovary of the postmenopausal woman. It contains few follicles and consists mainly of old corpora albicantia and corpora atretica cells. Most of the functional tissue has been replaced by connective-tissue fibres.

sensate-focus-oriented therapy the Masters and Johnson approach to sexual difficulties, which involves training sessions in which both Partners learn to think and feel sensually by Progressively touching, stroking, fondling, kissing, and massaging all Parts of their mate's body, with special attention to the erogenous zones. The purpose is to arouse the most exciting possible 96 stations in their partner and themselves. The therapy also includes a detailed history of each patient's attitudes and patterns, improvement in communication between the partners, reassurance and support, and prescribed practice at home.

sensuality unrestrained indulgence in the pleasures of the senses, particularly food and sex gratification of the 'carnal appetites.'

sensuous appealing to the senses, as in sensuous music, poetry, or painting. The term is also applied to a person with appreciates and enjoys experiences that involve the senses, including erotic stimulation.

Separate ova two or more ova released at the same time. Fertilization of separate ova results in dizygotic, or fraternal, twins. About 70 percent of twins are the result of multiple ovulation. Triplets or other multiple births also can result from separate ova. Studies indicate that the tendency to release separate ova at the same time is an inherited trait.

septate hymen a hymen that has an opening blocked only by a vertical fold of tissue in the middle.

septum a partition. The septum of the brain is associated with sexuality. It is part of the limbic system of the brain. Stimulation of the limbic system, and particularly the septum, results in erections and orgasms for monkeys and humans.

sequential pills a system of administering oral contraceptives in which pills containing only oestrogen are taken for 15 days. On the following 5 days, the woman takes pills containing both oestrogen and progestagen. The manufacturers note that this routine follows the natural pattern of female sex hormones more closely than in taking only pills containing both types of hormones.

serial monogamy a sequence of monogamous marriages; consecutive marriages, with divorce or annulment between, so that the individual is married to only one partner at a time. The term serial monogamy also applies to a form of courting behaviour in which young men and women remain faithful to each other as long as the relationship lasts. However, the relationship may be of short duration. One survey indicated that serial monogamists maintained a relationship for an average of a year or more but each had averaged four partners. Nearly half had experienced premarital sex as part of the relationship.

serosa an alternative term for the serous coat, which covers the uterus. It is derived from the peritoneum, a membrane that covers many of the pelvic structures.

serous cyst a large fluid-filled cyst of the ovary. It is grey to amber in colour and is named after the type of fluid, which resembles blood serum. A serous cyst of the ovary may grow to the size of an orange.

Sertoli cells the supporting cells of the seminiferous tubules in the testes. They are found between germinal cells and contain spermatids in their cytoplasm.

Sertoll-cells-only syndrome an alternative term for an abnormal condition of the testes in which only Sertoli cells are present and there is no germinal epithelium in the tubules.

sessile nodule a partial extrusion of sex chromatin material from the nucleus into the cytoplasm of a white blood cell of a female. The phenomenon, which is peculiar to females, is associated with the presence of Barr bodies in the white cells. If the chromatin material is completely extruded, it is called a drumstick appendage. The patterns of sex chromatin extrusion are representative of the sex chromosomal complements of the individuals.

17-ketosteroids substances produced in the adrenal cortex of both males and females. The 17-ketosteroids play an important role in sexual development and function as they are able to divert amino acids, the building blocks of proteins, into muscle mass and sex organs. The ketosteroids stimulate pubic-hair growth in adolescence, contribute to the enlargement of the penis and clitoris at puberty, and are responsible for much of the adolescent problem of acne.

sex the physical and psychological characteristics that distinguish between males and females; attributes that determine one's gender; also, the functions and processes involved in interoourse and procreation. In addition have sex means to have sexual intercourse, copulate.' The term is derived from the Latin word *sexus*, which appears to be related to *secare*, meaning to cut or to divide.

sex act any form of copulation or sexual intercourse, coitus.

sex addiction another term for sexual addiction.

sex after childbirth another term for postpartum intercourse.

sex-aggression rapist a rapist who associates violence and sadism with sex He usually has a history of antisocial and aggressive behaviour and may be impotent in sexual encounters with a woman unless the woman fights back. The violence itself is needed for his sexual arousal. Although the sex-aggression-fusion rapist is relatively rare, attacks by this type of person tend to be well publicized and result in more common forms of rape being overlooked or unreported.

Sexaholics Anonymous an American organization of individuals who consider them selves addicted to sex and who conduct Periodic meetings to discuss their preoccupation with sexual matters. Patterned, after Alcoholics Anonymous, Sexaholics Anonymous is organized into local chapters, Members include persons who have risked jobs, family, and friends to maintain expensive contacts with prostitutes, massage pariours, and pornographic shops.

sex aids another term for erotic aids.

sex and alcohol intake of alcoholic drinks as a means of increasing the sex drive or enhancing sexual performance. Studies show that modest amounts may help people overcome anxiety, fear or inhibition, and enable them to 'relax and enjoy it! Large amounts, however, have been found to decrease or even eliminate the man's capacity to achieve or maintain an erection, and the woman's ability to have an orgasm. Alcohol may also impair judgment and open the way to sexual activity that may be later regretted; under its influence, contraceptives may be forgotten and unwanted pregnancy may result.

sex and disability the view that individuals affected by severe physical disability such as cerebral palsy, paraplegia, and multiple sclerosis, have the right to and, in most cases, the capacity for sexual gratification—and in some instances can have children of their own. Even in cases where they cannot achieve full orgasm, they are almost always capable of some form of sexual pleasure and excitement, provided they have the opportunity to experiment with every possible form of stimulation: masturbation, oral sex, and homosexual relationships where desired, plus any variation in position that works, or any artificial aid such as a vibrator, or even a third party acting as an assistant.

sex and social class general differences in sexual attitudes and behaviour observed on different socioeconomic levels. Using education as an indicator, Kinsey found that single males with some higher education relied more heavily on masturbation, deep kissing, petting, and nocturnal emissions, and less heavily on relations with prostitutes and homosexual contacts than males with less education. Highly educated men are also generally more responsive to the sexual needs of their wives than are the less well-educated, and more likely to believe that a woman's sexual gratification is as important as a man's.

sex apparatus the internal and external sexual organs as well as the glands that produce the sexual products or that stimulate or control the functions of the sexual organs or the development of secondary sex characteristics.

sex appeal the capacity to arouse sexual interest and desire. This is largely a matter of personal taste and cultural pattern. However, generally speaking, people in Western society are particularly responsive to athletic, muscular, somewhat aggressive men, and relatively slim women with slightly oversized breasts, shapely legs and buttocks, careful makeup, flowing hair, and revealing or pro, vocative clothes. In certain non-Western societies the sources of sex appeal are extremely varied, including such features as gigantic buttocks, pendulous breasts, flattened heads, protruding navels, crossed eyes, blackened teeth, artificially stretched necks, and scarred or tattooed bodies.

sex-appropriate behaviour behaviour that is considered suited to one's sex.

sex assignment identification of an individual as male, female, pseudohermaphrodite, or hermaphrodite, on the basis of physical characteristics. Transsexuals do not accept their sex assignment, feeling that they are victims of a mistake of nature, and some of them may request sex-change operations.

sex-blind a term applied to US state laws that Prohibit discrimination between the sexes, such as insurance laws that prohibit differences in rates based on sex.

sex centre of the brain a term sometimes applied to a small area at the base of the brain which is believed to control the sex drive and various sexual functions, including the ovulation cycle in the female and ejaculation in the male. Its principal component is the Pituitary gland, the 'master gland' that Programs not only the sex glands but every other gland in the body. Studies have also suggested that damage in this area may be one of the causes of nymphomania and satyriasis on the one hand, and impotence and diminished sex interest on the other.

sex change the alteration of a patient's external sex organs through surgery and hormone treatments with the aim of making them conform as closely as possible to the physical structures of the opposite sex. The procedure is typically Performed on male transsexuals, and occasionally on female transsexuals. Both male and female transsexuals are convinced that they have been trapped in the wrong body, and insist that they are meant to be members of the opposite sex physically, emotionally, and mentally.

The male-to-female operation is usually preceded by a year of psychiatric evaluation and counselling, accompanied by hormone injections and cross-dressing. During the surgical procedure, the penis and testes are removed and labia and vagina are constructed. In the female-to-male procedure, skin from the abdomen and labia are used to construct a penis and scrotum. The requests for male-to-female sex changes average about 20 to 1 in frequency over requests by females to be changed into males.

sex characteristics visible features associated with gender identity and reproduction.

sex chromatin a dark mass representing the X chromosome that can be observed in a human cell that has been stained with a particular dye for study under a microscope. The X chromosome must be inactive to absorb the stain. Therefore, only cells of a female will reveal the chromatin presence by this test. A normal male, with one X and one Y chromosome will not have body cells with one extra, inactive X chromosome and thus will not have cells that show the stain. Although the female has two X chromosomes, only, one will be active. A male body cell showing sex chromatin would suggest that the male had a chromosome abnormality, such as Klinefelter's syndrome, with an XXY or XXYY chromosome complement. A female with a multiple X chromosome abnormality, such as an XXX or XXXX complement, probably would have body cells that would show sex chromatin in two or more areas when stained for the test.

sex chromosomes the chromosomes that determine the gender of an individual. A normal human female possesses two X chromosomes, although only one of the X chromosomes is active. The normal human male has one X and one Y chromosome. The function of the Y chromosome apparently is to code the embryonic molecules necessary to produce male sex hormones. A normal female complement of sex chromosomes is identified as XX, and the normal male set is indicated as XY. It is difficult if not impossible to determine precisely which of the human sex chromosomes is actually an X or a Y chromosome. The X chromosome bears an almost exact resemblance to any of the 14 chromosomes in the second row of a standard karyotype, and the chromosome used to represent the Y sex chromosome may be interchangeable with either chromosome 21 or 22, which have the same size and shape.

sex-chromosome aberrations any variation from the normal male complement of an XY set of sex chromosomes or deviation from the normal female complement of an XX set of sex chromosomes in addition to the 22 pairs of autosomes. One-of the most common aberrations is Klinefelter's syndrome, in which a male has one, two, or three extra X chromosomes. The extra chromosomes alter the individual's sexual characteristics in varying degrees, but the usual manifestations include hypogenitalism and infertility. The person with Klinefelter's syndrome also may have a deficiency of some male secondary sexual characteristics. But in many cases, the condition is not revealed until the person has married and his infertility has resulted in a visit to a medical specialist in an effort to find the reason for being sterile. An extra X chromosome in a female is even more likely to go unnoticed because fertility would not be affected. There is a possibility that the female with extra X chromosomes might be mentally retarded, the only consistent manifestation in sex-chromosome disorders. In fact, a female with as many as five X chromosomes could appear quite normal in so far as secondary sexual characteristics are concerned. The woman with three or more X chromosomes often is identified as a 'superfemale' or 'metafemale.'

A male with extra Y chromosomes, similarly might appear physically as a 'supermale' with normal sexual development and a body size above average. Except for possible mental retardation and aberrant behaviour, the only noticeable defect could be a lack of good muscular coordination. A female sexchromosome aberration that is characterized by abnormal physical features is Turner's syndrome, a condition in which the individual receives only one sex chromosome, an X chromosome.

sex counselling guidance provided to an individual or couple by a sex therapist, social worker, psychiatrist, or doctor on such questions as conception, family planning, infertility, fear of failure in performance, unresponsiveness, sexual anatomy and physiology, and techniques of intercourse.

sex determination the random sorting of male gametes, or spermatozoa, containing either an X sex chromosome or a Y sex chromosome as they approach a female gamete, or ovum, which always will contain only an X chromosome. The spermatozoon that finally merges with the ovum will determine the sex of the new individual by forming either an XX, or female, combination of sex chromosomes, or an XY, or male, combination. Regardless of external sexual characteristics, the sex of the individual in adult life will be determined by the type of gonad, that develops in the person. Genetically, a person with ovaries will be classified as female, and an individual with testes will be considered a male.

sex differences overall differences, or alleged differences, between males and females on primary sex characteristics, secondary sex characteristics, personality characteristics, social roles, type and level of intelligence, motor-development skills and aptitudes, interests and values, emotional adjustment, and life expectancy, as well as differences in sexual development and behaviour, including sexuality in infancy and childhood, age for entering puberty, frequency of masturbation, frequency of orgasm, and the comparative ages for the peak and diminution of sexual activity.

sex differentiation the process of developing anatomical features typical of male or female sex, or, in rare cases, hermaphroditism. These characteristics are genetically determined at the time of fertilization, but do not begin to appear externally until the seventh or eighth week.

sex discrimination discrimination against an individual or group of individuals on the basis of sex, especially in regard to the type of job, remuneration, and opportunities for tenure or promotion. Currently the term also applies to discrimination against male and sometimes female homosexuals not only in the job market but in holding public office, membership in social-or political organizations, and clubs.

sex doll a life-sized, inflatable doll with somewhat exaggerated sexual features, including large breasts, an open mouth, a full head of hair, and a relatively realistic vagina and anus as well as pubic hair. Typically, these dolls are sold to men who suffer from shyness, loneliness, or physical handicap or to sailors or others who have no immediate access to women. For women, sex dolls such as a male torso with an inflatable penis have also become available.

sex dreams an alternative term for nocturnal emissions, which usually occur during erotic male dreaming. Sex dreams also occur among women, but are less common. A Kinsey study found about 4 percent of women experience nocturnal orgasms while dreaming and most such events happen among older single women.

sex drive the primary, probably instinctual, urge for sexual gratification. On the average, the impulse reaches its peak in the late teens among males and in the 30s among females. Although both sexes maintain an interest in sexual activity throughout their lives, by the age of 50 the average man is satisfied with two orgasms per week, and beginning in the 50s and 60s the average woman experiences a slight decline in sex drive, and is usually less Preoccupied with sex than in her earlier years. Unlike other primary drives such as hunger and thirst survival of the individual does not depend on the sex drive, though survival of the species does. Also, in contrast to lower species, the human sex drive is less seasonal, less dependent upon an oestrous cycle, more varied in expression, and aroused by a wider range of stimuli.

sex during menstruation intercourse during menstrual flow. Although the practice is discouraged by some cultures and individuals, a Masters and Johnson study found that only 10 percent of women object to sexual activity during menstruation, mainly for religious or aesthetic reasons. Of those approving of the practice, it was indicated that orgasm during menstruation helped expel the menstrual fluid at a rapid rate, thereby reducing the pain and discomfort often associated with menstruation. In most societies intercourse is forbidden or frowned upon during menstruation, for example, among Hindus. The Naayar of India go farther and believe that man who has intercourse with a menstruating woman is likely to become impotent

sex during pregnancy a term referring to the advisability of continuing intercourse during pregnancy. Specialists usually allow their Patients to continue sex relations until approximately the seventh month if there is no discharge or pain. As pregnancy advances, some modification of coital position will be necessary. They also assure their Patients that intercourse will not harm the baby or cause a miscarriage.

sex education instruction on the physical, psychological, and behavioural aspects of sex, given in a classroom setting, but also through books and other publications. Formal sex education is designed to supplement or correct information and misinformation imparted by parents, peers, and the mass media.

sex experimentation among children, the tendency to explore each other's bodies, to, imitate intercourse before being capable of achieving it, or in some cases to fondle, kiss, masturbate, or perform fellatio or cunnilingus. Among teenagers all forms of foreplay (necking, petting) and many forms of intercourse may be tried, as well as variations they have seen or read about in magazines, such as erotic bondage, flagellation, bestiality, and experimenting with the effects of drugs of various kinds. Among adults all these may be tried, also other variations such as group sex, partner swapping, trial marriage, and open marriage.

sex fiend a colloquial term for a sex offender who commits sadistic acts of the most extreme kind, such as a series of rapes, mutilation of the sex organs of victims, or homicide after sexual assault, Many of these offenders are psychotic.

sex hormones chemical 'messengers' that control the sexual and reproductive processes. The primary sources are the pituitary gland, the ovaries, the testes, and the adrenal cortex.

sex hospitality a sexual practice in which a man's wife (or sometimes daughter) is placed at the disposal of a male guest as a gesture of friendship and hospitality. The custom has been found in many parts of the world, including Africa, Siberia, Polynesia, Alaska,˘ and the Aleutian Islands.

sex hygiene measures taken to insure clean, healthy, well-functioning sexual organs. These include washing with water (avoiding the use of scented soap or sprays just before intercourse, because they destroy exciting sexual odours) and Precautions for the prevention of venereal disease. Women need to take special Precautions to maintain cleanliness during menstruation, and also need periodic, smear tests and gynaecological examinations, with attention to discharges, lumps, and bleeding. In addition, good sex hygiene involves general fitness, because sexual activity requires considerable expenditure of energy, especially if it is vigorous and prolonged.

sexing piece an older term for penis.

sex initiative taking the lead in suggesting intercourse or other sexual activity, either openly or indirectly, In Victorian times men were generally expected to take the initiative, although women might sometimes take the lead by using their 'wiles.' However, because women have achieved a greater measure of social equality in the present era, they are far more likely to take the sexual initiative than in the past sexism a pattern of discrimination against an individual (usually a female) or group stemming from prejudicial beliefs and attitudes. Examples are 'A woman's place is in the home,' 'Women can't stand up to competition,' 'Women are the weaker sex,' 'Women should not engage in body-contact sports,' or 'Women are too emotional for executive positions.'

sexless gonad the embryonic gonad at 6 weeks after conception. The sex has been determined genetically at conception, but at 6 weeks the structure is an indifferent sex gland that could be either a male or female gonad.

sex-limited character a trait that is normally expressed in only one sex, for example, the tendency to balding among men.

sex-linked character a characteristic that is determined by genes of one of the sex chromosomes. The term applies mainly to recessive traits located on the X chromosome. For this reason, men are more likely to be affected than women. In women, the trait will be masked by a dominant gene for the characteristic in most instances, whereas the Y chromosome will lack a dominant gene for the trait.

sex maniac a popular term for an individual, who is preoccupied with sexual satisfaction and sexual exploits, including such variations as voyeurism, exhibitionism, a history of seducing a maximum number of men or women, as well as more malignant behaviour such as murder, mutilation, and intercourse with corpses for sexual gratification.

sex manuals handbooks written for the explicit purpose of imparting sex information and promoting sex education. The first handbooks were probably the early pillow books,' but the first manuals that could be called modem were Dr. Albutt's The Wife's Handbook and Marie Stopes' Married Love.

sex-negative a term referring mainly to social institutions, to a society's rituals, religions, and so on that restrict sexual expression, For example, Christianity has often been called the most sex-negative of all religions.

sex object a person, animal, or inanimate object towards which sexual impulses are directed. The term is often used in a derogatory sense, because many women resent being treated primarily as objects for stimulation and gratification.

sex offender an individual who commits sex offences that are punishable by law. The term includes milder offences stemming from neurotic trends, such as voyeurism, as well as more severe offences such as forcible rape, stemming from a severe personality disturbance and possibly from a chromosomal disorder. Contrary to popular opinion, the typical convicted sex offender is undersexed and severely inhibited rather than oversexed. The majority are in their late teens or early twenties, and 50 to 60 percent are unmarried.

sexologist a professional worker who has been trained to engage in research, therapy, or educational programmes in the field of human sexuality.

sexology the scientific study of sexuality and sexual behaviour, including sexual relationships, sexual practices, sexual disorders, sexual anatomy and physiology, and sex education. The field draws its content from studies of human and animal behaviour, psychology, psychiatry, anthropology, medicine, sociology, education, and the law.

sex play an expression referring to (a) children's exploratory activities such as the doctor game; (b) children's play that has a sexual tinge, such as hair pulling and wrestling; (c) foreplay preceding intercourse; (d) erotic activities short of intercourse, such as necking and petting; and (e) masturbatory activities, or 'playing with oneself.'

sex prediction the ability to forecast or select in advance the gender of an offspring. A number of techniques are used, including intercourse before ovulation to increase the likelihood that a girl will be conceived or immediately after ovulation to increase chances for a boy, or use of an acid douche before intercourse to increase the chances of producing a female offspring or an alkali douche to improve the likelihood of conceiving a boy. Amniocentesis can be used to find out the sex of a child before delivery; however, the results are usually not available until the 17th or 18th week of a pregnancy. Physicians in China reported a technique of accurately predicting the sex of an unborn child 47 days after conception by scraping cells from the cervix of the mother. Many Old Wives' tales have been used over the centuries to explain predetermined sex selection. One of the oldest is the notion that one testicle contains sperm producing only girls and the other holds sperm that produces only boys.

sex ratio the proportion of male and female infants born in a given population. The usual frequency is about 106 males to 100 females. Later in life, the rate of premature male deaths usually exceeds that of female so that eventually the ratio shifts and women outnumber men of the same age group.

sex roannouncement an announcement to members of the family and community that a child first identified in birth announcements as a boy has now been correctly identified as a girl, or vice versa. Bemuse external genitalia at birth are sometimes misidentified as to gender, resulting in an incorrect birth announcement, a later announcement is made to correct the information.

sex reassignment change in sex assignment resulting from a sex-change operation. If the operation is a success, the male may feel more comfortable as a female, and perform sexually as a female, though he will not be able to conceive and reproduce. Females may become, to all intents and purposes, male except that it-will not be possible to impregnate a woman.

sex-reassignment operation an alternative term for sex-change operation, or surgery in which a male is transformed into a female, or vice versa.

sex relations a broad term for any physical relationship between two or more people that serves the purpose of arousing or satisfying the sexual impulse, ranging from necking and petting to all forms of intercourse. Sex relations include the exploratory sexual behaviour of children as well as premarital, extramarital, and marital sex.

sex research studies of sexual behaviour that can be documented in large populations, as distinguished from anecdotal information based on observations of a few individual subjects. Because of widely varied sexual behaviour of individuals, data based on observations of a few cases can be misleading.

sex reversal the procedures involved in transforming a man into a woman or a woman into a man, with appropriate surgery, administration of sex hormones, and psychological counselling.

sex rituals rites and ceremonies prescribed by various societies, and religions as a means of celebrating or controlling sex activities. Examples are ritual baths required by the Hindus and Hebrews after menstruation; ritual intercourse performed by the Asian Lepchas in a special position 3, 7, and 21 days after the birth of a baby; exchange of wives conceived as a purification rite among the Murngin of Australia; and the requirement, in several African societies, that the boy have sex with a married woman as part of his initiation ceremony.

sex-role Inventory any psychological test in which the individuals rate themselves on personality characteristics indicative of their sex role.

sex-role stereotypes fixed, oversimplified patterns of sexual behaviour and attitudes as defined in a given society, such as the traditional concepts of males as relatively unemotional, rational, decisive, strong, and brave; and of females as highly emotional, illogical, weak, dependent, and unfit for participation in the rough-and-tumble world outside the home. An example of a nontraditional stereotype is that of the androgynous sex role, which combines features of both male and female.

sex selection the process of determining before coitus the sex of the offspring. It is claimed by Landrum Shettles of Columbia University that an alkaline douche (made with baking soda) before intercourse will increase the chances that a boy will be conceived, while an acid douche, made with vinegar, will increase the odds for conception of a girl, Professor Shettles also recommends coitus before ovulation for couples hoping for a girl and sexual intercourse after ovulation for those wishing for a boy.

sex shows live performances that feature nudity or sexual activity. Such performances, are said to date from the days of the Roman emperors Tiberius and Caligula, and have been associated with many royal courts since that time. In India travelling entertainers performed almost incredible feats of sexual gymnastics. Private erotic theatres existed in the Western world from time to time, and during the 19th century scenes of copulation, lesbian ads, and bestiality were enacted in brothels. Many modern Western performances such as striptease and several theatrical productions belong in this general category.

sex skin the minor lips of the sexually excited woman, which become progressively more pink and red during the plateau phase of the sexual response cycle. If erotic stimulation continues, the lips become more swollen and engorged with blood, orgasm is usually inevitable. The term is also applied to the sexually sensitive area of the skin adjacent to the female genitals.

sex statistics the quantified data of sex research. Although statistics are an accepted research device, the interpretation of results, can be misleading, particularly when expressed in terms such as 'average' or 'percent' or 'normal.' Many persons tend to confuse average with 'normal' and regard sexual behaviour that is not average as 'abnormal' which is not the intention of the statistical report.

sex-stereotyped play childhood games and play activities that are traditionally associated with either male or female sex roles, such as boys playing with action toys or in competitive sports while girls play with dolls.

sex stereotyping the development of a sexual typology based on behaviour and attitudes that are considered by society to be appropriate for males and females, such as the expectation (now questioned) that all girls and women have a special interest in homemaking activities, or for boys and men to be more interested in muscular activities than women (which is also being questioned).

sexual aberrations any deviations from normal or typical sexual behaviour, especially those associated with mental or emotional disorders. Examples are sexual sadism, sexual masochism, paedophilia, fetishism, exhibitionism, voyeurism, transvestism, zoophilia, coprophilia, and necrophilia.

sexual ability the capacity to become sexually excited and, in particular, to achieve orgasm. In the male, sexual ability depends on the capacity to achieve and maintain erection, and in the female, the capacity to become aroused when the erogenous zones are stroked or manipulated. Most people of both sexes are also capable of becoming sexually excited by dreams, fantasies, films, or pictures, without physical contact of any kind.

sexual abnormality sexual behaviour that does not conform to the accepted expressions of sexuality within a given culture or community. It is important for an individual to understand what is considered as normal sexual behaviour to avoid feelings of guilt about his or her own fantasies and practices, which may not actually deviate from those of other persons in the culture or community even though they are not openly sanctioned by the more conservative members of the group.

sexual abstinence refraining from sexual activity temporarily or permanently. Examples of temporary abstinence are during menstruation or late pregnancy, before marriage, or during certain religious celebrations. Lifelong abstinence is required as a means of expressing holiness among Catholic nuns and priests.

sexual abuse physical injury administered for the purpose of sexual arousal or gratification in the abuser or, in some cases, in the victim. Milder forms are pinching, slapping, and squeezing; more extreme forms are whipping, beating, cutting, biting, and, in rare instances, mutilation of the sex organs or other parts of the body.

sexual activity a general term covering any kind of behaviour, such as petting, flagellation, masturbation, and intercourse, whose purpose is to produce sexual excitement.

sexual addiction according to recent sex therapists, a pattern of excessive, repetitive sexual activity that resembles addiction to alcohol or drugs in providing relief from feelings of anxiety or worthlessness. For some individuals, possibly one in 12, sex becomes an all-consuming compulsion pursued at the expense of marriage, career, or family life. An increasing number of sex therapists are dealing with this problem, and a number of self-help groups modelled after Alcoholics Anonymous have been formed.

sexual advances any deliberate attempt to arouse sexual interest or response in another individual. Sexual advances vary widely, and include indirect approaches such as smiling, winking, firmly holding the other person's hand when introduced, inviting the other person to share drinks, as well as more direct approaches, such as stroking, caressing, suggesting 'Let's go to my place,' and making a direct 'proposition.'

sexual affinity a strong sexual attraction between two individuals of the opposite or the same sex.

sexual-aim rapist a rapist who is truly sexually motivated and uses only as much force as is necessary to achieve intercourse. He may have fantasies of his victims falling in love with him after he has demonstrated his sexual prowess.

sexual anaesthesia an inability to experience sexual feeling; frigidity.

sexual analism sexual intercourse in which the penis is inserted into the anus of the partner. Except for occasional experiments, the practice, also known as sodomy, is seldom performed in heterosexual contacts.

sexual apathy a negative attitude towards sexual relations, ranging from indifference and listlessness to active revulsion, for an extended period—despite propitious circumstances and a willing partner. The precise reasons may be hard to fathom, but apathy is often based on a distasteful or painful experience, a monotonous and unimaginative approach on the part of one or both partners, the pressure of business or home responsibilities, preoccupation with other interests and events, excessive demands by the partner, chronic fatigue, general depression, or unconscious conflicts over sex.

sexual appetite the need, or the desire, for sexual gratification. The sex urge has been found to vary greatly from person to person and time to time.

sexual athlete a man or woman whose sex life is

governed by quantity more than quality, and who engages in practically every conceivable coital position and variation, even the most outlandish. To sexual athletes, sex is more of a game or sport than an expression of affection.

sexual attitudes attitudes towards sex and behaviour as influenced by such factors as family relationships and upbringing, and the demands, expectations, and sexual ethics of the particular culture and subculture in which one lives. There are wide cultural differences around the world; for example, in a study of 158 societies, 70 percent were tolerant of premarital intercourse, but not of adulterous relationships; in societies where sexual expression among women is approved or encouraged, they are as uninhibited and active as men; and in American society, attitudes towards virginity at marriage have changed dramatically in the past generation.

sexual attraction the capacity to elicit sexual interest through a provocative manner or exciting physical features, such as full lips and shapely breasts, legs and buttocks in women, and an athletic build in men. In many cases reputation as a skilled lover also increases attraction. Various societies have developed unique ways of increasing sexual attraction.

sexual awakening a period of psychological change that accompanies pubescence. It is usually marked by changes in attitudes, emotions, and interests that are more appropriate for this stage of approaching sexual maturity. It also is a period in which physical experimentation, including increased masturbation, occurs.

sexual behaviour the sexual activity of an individual

as observed by others, as distinguished from a subjective or inner perspective on one's own sexual acts. Other characteristics of sexual behaviour may include conscious, unconscious or innate, or socially determined components, with biological, psychological, and developmental influences.

Behavioural assessment is more important than behaviour therapy. Anyone who has struggled with the application of behavioural techniques to complex behavioural problems is aware that the most difficult part of this endeavor is the development of adequate behavioural measures. Once adequate measures are developed, therapy is often a matter of applying the usual and standard techniques of selective, positive reinforcement or modeling, as even a cursory look at the literature.

The notion that assessment will determine the nature of therapy is not limited to the behavioural approach. Bergin and Strupp note that more accurate assessment of various problems comprising any diagnostic category will lead to the construction of specific treatments aimed at specific components of a problem.

Yet the development of the area of behavioural assessment has lagged behind the development of new behaviour therapies. In our headlong rush to develop new treatment in 1960s, assessment efforts by which we judged the adequacy of these treatments were often no better than an answer a patient would give to the question, "How are you feeling now?" In some cases actual behavioural measures were utilized, but more often than not these measures were tangential to the behavioural problems that brought the patient for treatment. Although this book begins to address the problem of the underdevelopment of behavioural assessment and the communication of recent developments in this area to practicing clinicians,, it will come as no surprise that there are many more questions than answers concerning procedures and techniques used in behavioural assessment, particularly in clinical settings. Against this background, the behavioural assessment of sexual behaviour is particularly interesting since many of the problems and issues confronting the field of assessment today are illustrated when one attempts to assess sexual behaviour.

Major issues to be discussed here include the relationship of self-report to behavioural and physiological response systems in the assessment of sexual behaviour. A second issue involves the use of contrived situations versus naturalistic observation in the assessment of all three components of sexual behaviour. The necessity of assessing early components in the chain of sexual arousal will also be discussed. In addition, the complexity of sexual behaviour, discovered in the last few years, has led to the conclusion that many of our labels for sexual behaviour are inadequate. In sexual deviation, for example, no client is the same. Each has some combination of behavioural excesses and defects, and each requires individual assessment. Data presented later in this chapter will illustrate that people supposedly falling in the category of one label used in sexual deviation, such as pedophilia, may actually be more different from one another than any two people who do not share this label. Similarly, it is not useful to talk about sexual inadequacy such as orgasmic dysfunction or impotence unless one is using these terms in a purely descriptive manner, because these terms do not carry the precision to lead to specific interventions. Finally, in deviations in gender role the categorization of males as "effeminate" or females as "masculine" grossly oversimplifies the enormous complexities of gender identity and deviations in gender role as well as their implications for treatment.

Following this discussion is a description of the three major components of sexual behaviour: sexual arousal, heterosexual social skills (heterosocial skills), and gender identity or gender role deviations.

The importance of assessing all three response systems is one of the more important developments in recent years and appears repeatedly throughout this book. The lack of relationship among the verbal, the motororic, and the physiological response systems is well known by now. In the assessment of most behavioural problems, however, differential importance is attributed to these response systems depending on one's general approach or orientation to the problems. Certainly the term *behavioural assessment* indicates a preference for assessment of the behavioural or motoric response system. Many behavioural clinicians assess self-report only if direct measurements of behavior are unobtainable. Until recent years, the difficulty in measuring sexual behaviour directly forced a reliance on verbal or self-report measures.

The tendency to ignore self-report since the development of reliable physiological measures of sexual arousal is not consistent with the discovery of three independent response systems and could even the dangerous. This tendency in behavioural assessment of sexual behaviour or other clinical problems ignores the fact that self-report *is* behaviour and therefore is just as important as direct observation of physiological arousal or heterosexual social skills, or even direct observation of sexual interactions. This notion is at variance with the approach that categorizes self-report measures as indirect measures of behaviour. Because self-report of sexual problems may or may not correlate with the other response systems, it is inaccurate to call these measures indirect.

The fact is that there are several different types of self-report measures used in the assessment or sexual problems or other clinical problems, some of which may correlate with behavioural or physiological response systems better that others. For example, self-monitoring of sexual behaviour, such as reports of number of orgasms reached during sexual interactions, may correlate highly with directly observed behaviour under certain conditions. Rating scale measures of subjective discomfort during sexual behaviour may correlate poorly with physiological or behavioural measures of sexual behaviour. For example, in a recent study, the sexual responding of six heterosexual and six homosexual males was assessed while they were watching several erotic movies, including a movie depicting homosexual interaction. Penile circumference, subjective reports of sexual arousal, and attitudinal ratings of "pleasantness" were measured. Heterosexual males reported the homosexual movie a distinctly unpleasant but demonstrated penile erection averaging 20 percent of a full erection and also reported being sexually aroused. The point of interest here is the split between two different self-report measures of sexual functioning.

In general, self-report correlates fairly well with objective measures of arousal, at least in nonpatient populations. In the study cited above, a self report measure of arousal correlated 0.64 with measures of erection across all subjects and attitudinal reports of "pleasantness" correlated 0.55. Attitudinal measures and self-reports of arousal correlated 0.82. Geer notes that Heiman reports similar correlations for "normal" women between self-report of arousal and genital responding of 0.54 to 0.60. As Geer points out, this is a higher correlation than is found between self-report and other physiological responding.

In a patient population, however, Hoon, Wincze, and Hoon noted that sexually "normal" women and sexually dysfunctional women subjectively rated their arousal as similar during an erotic movie. But sexually dysfunctional women were not aroused compared to the normal group, suggesting a split between objective and subjective measures in this patient population. A more careful exploration of the different varieties of self-report of sexual behaviour and their relationship to one another as well as to treatment outcome is an important area for future research.

Whenever the results of future research, one can make a strong case that in the assessment of sexual behaviour in the clinic, self-report measures are at present more important than behavioural or physiological measures. This rather unusual statement is true because sexual problems that one confronts in the clinic occur almost entirely in adult populations. These patients are typically voluntary outpatients who report that they have a sexual problem such as a deviant arousal pattern or sexually dysfunctional behaviour. Self-report of these problems, then becomes the only necessary criterion for entry into treatment. This differs markedly form the way in which institutionalized people or other patients in closed settings enter into treatment, a process that usually begins with direct observation of some unacceptable behaviour. Similarly, self-assessment of progress is often the major criterion for terminating the intervention. Accurate depiction of patterns of sexual arousal that are reliably and independently measured and that demonstrate continued existence of a sexual problem will not keep a patient in treatment if he reports that he feels better and has recovered from the problem. When this happens, treatment is over. This fairly common occurrence in the clinic highlights the importance of understanding the relationship of self-report to other response systems and to outcome at follow-up. A further understanding of the variables controlling the reporting of different aspects of self-report is particularly important in cases when self-report diverges from behavioural or physiological measures. This is a common occurrence, as demonstrated in several cases described later.

Despite the relatively high correlation between self-report and physiological response in nonpatient populations, experience indicates that it is very common for divergences in the various response systems to occur during the assessment of sexual behaviour in patient populations as in the Hoon et al. study described above. There seem to be at least two reason for this. In our culture sexual behaviour is still a rather sensitive subject, difficult for many people to describe. Second, recent findings from our laboratories indicate that even patients who seem very willing to report their sexual behaviour as accurately as possible produce reports that diverge from objectively measured sexual arousal.

A patient who came to one of our outpatient clinics several years ago with complaints of anxiety and some depression provides an example of the difficulty in pinpointing sexual problems. Subsequent careful interviewing in a behavioural context revealed that the anxiety or feeling of uneasiness seemed to be correlated with specific people in his environment, but it was difficult to determine why. After some further discussion, it was decided there were some general social skill deficits, and a treatment program was begun to deal with these interpersonal problems. This patient came regularly for his appointments, weekly at first and then once every two weeks, for almost a year. Although some improvement was evident, the patient continued to report general feelings of unhappiness, anxiety, and depression at intensities that were unchanged since he had begun treatment, yet he continued to come, paying the standard fee each session. It was only by chance, during a routine reevaluation, that the patient finally blurted out that he had overwhelming homosexual attraction and arousal that was "the reason" for his difficulty in interpersonal situations. When asked why he had continued to come to treatment sessions all year long, paying $40.00 an hour, without mentioning what was really bothering him, he simply said that he had wanted to report these attractions all year but was unable to bring himself to do so.

Similar situations have arisen on several occasions in our clinics where presumably there is some expertise in identifying and interviewing sexual problems. This illustrates the scope of the problem and highlights the importance of the initial interview. In view of the fact that one cannot begin to assess sexual behaviour in voluntary adult patients unless the patients first report the presence of a sexual problem, the manner in which one approaches sexual behaviour in the initial interview is very important. In our view the problem in obtaining such information most often comes about when young clinicians communicate to patients in subtle ways that they are more uneasy gathering information in the sexual area than in other areas o the patient's life. If the clinician communicates that he is sensitive about sexual matters, it is very difficult for the patient. The best approach is a direct approach in which inquiries about sexual matters are treated mush the same as inquiries about other aspects of the patient's behaviour. If one suspects that the patient is having difficulty reporting sexual behaviour, it is helpful to return to the subject later in the interview. At that time the clinician can remind the patient that some people have difficulty talking about sexual material but that accurate reporting of such behaviour is necessary to determine how best to help the patient. One must often move from the clinical language of sexual functioning to colloquialisms peculiar to the patient's own cultural setting. Interviewing procedures will be discussed further in the section on self-report measures.

A second example of the discrepancy between verbal report and behaviour occurs when the patient is perfectly willing to discuss his problem but seems unable to report the functional relationships accurately. It seems as though he really doesn't know what his problem is. In describing a patient with whom this problem occurred, I will also describe what I think is one of the more sophisticated approaches to assessment of sexual arousal. This approach uses direct measures of genital arousal, and I will illustrate its use in a typical, functionally analytic manner. The procedure was devised by Abel and is one we have been using in our laboratory for several years. Essentially, the method involves presenting sexual cues by audiotapes, which are then played back to the patient. While he listens to the tape, the erection responses on the read-out are observed. New audio tapes are then made, enlarging on the content that was correlated with penile responses. The new tape, in turn, will occasion further erections, usually larger than those noted on the first tape. Finally, the content of the tape correlated with the larger erections is once again elaborated on after considerable discussion with the patient. What emerges is an audiotape that is highly erotic to the patient undergoing assessment. This approach will described again in the section on assessing male sexual arousal. This method of establishing functional relationships between specific audio cues and erection responses can uncover patterns of arousal of which the subject is unaware. Such was the case with the patient who is described in the following paragraph.

The patient was a 22-year-old male who reported being very sexually aroused by white or brown, open-toed sandals. This pattern of arousal had been bothering him for approximately two years. In his detailed description he also reported fantasies of kissing the girl's feet and even smelling the girl's feet to see how sexy they were. De denied, however, that the woman's foot along was erotic and noted that the open-toed sandal was the key ingredient. Using the audiotape method, the first tape described an interaction with such a sandal, based on his report of what was erotic:

"You are in a room, in a room with a girl, she's got some sandals on, you see her sandals there. She's very attractive, you see her sandals, the white kind. You see them on her feet there, see the strap between her toes. She's got very pretty feet. You are looking at the white sandals there, very pretty, see how fit her fee, going in between her toes there, going in between her toes. See the leather there with plastic in between her toes, very attractive, white, very attractive, white leather sandals, open-toed, very attractive and white. See them on her, on her feet there, very attractive, and you see the shoes, sandal, white sandals, as you are walking over, and youre feeing the sandal, very white, you can feel it in your hands, the sandal, very white, holding it, you can feel the material."

Surprisingly, this scene generated very little arousal, only on the order of 20 percent. another tape was developed, excluding mention of the sandal but describing in some detail the girl's foot.

"Your are in a room with a girl and you are looking over at her, looking over at her, and you see her feet. She's really got beautiful feet, she's got sandals on, but you are looking at her feet, really beautiful feet, soft skin, very soft skin, very attractive feet, and you are starting to move over there towards her. She's just kind of playing with her sandals there, they drop to the ground. You come over and she's very willing to let you play with her feet, to hold her feet, caress them. You have your hands on her feet now, you are licking her feet, you can smell her feet, you are licking her feet. She wants you to do that, she wants you to feel her feet there, get a hold of her foot in your hands, you are licking her foot, kissing it, it's very, very sexy smelling. Really sexy smelling, she really wants you to hold her foot there. You feel it, you feel the smooth skin, very smooth, smooth skin on her foot, very attractive. You're just kind of holding her foot there, kissing her foot, her, holding it and kissing it. She's really turned on. Holding her foot she's really turned on by it. She's really turned on, holding her foot. You're really, really enjoying it. Feeling the skin on her foot, holding her foot, feeling the skin there, very smooth, very smooth skin."

This description generated 75 percent of a full erection. These data suggested that the foot rather than the sandal was he erotic cue. To confirm this, the patient listened to subsequent tapes containing references only to sandals. The data also supported the supposition that the girl's foot was the erotic object rather than the sandal, as the patient had reported. The discrepancy here was between a physiological measure of arousal and reports of arousal. When this discrepancy was discussed with the patient, he changed his verbal report to agree with the physiological findings.

Differences between verbal report and physiological assessment of arousal in the assessment of sexual behaviour can easily be produced in the laboratory. Several years ago we collected data during an experiment that examined the role of expectancy in an aversive procedure—covert sensitization. In covert sensitization the sexually arousing scene, as described by the therapist, is paired in imagination with noxious scenes such as nausea and vomiting or other aversive scenes taken directly from the patient's experiences. Both arousal, as measured by penile circumference changes, and self-report of arousal were assessed. During the first phase the sexually arousing scene was presented without the noxious scene. The subject relaxed and imagined a sexually arousing scene, but the instructions indicated that this would make them better, that is, less aroused. They were told that relaxing would "counteract" the arousal. When covert sensitization was administered, the patients were told that this procedure would actually make them more aroused owning to an increase in general tension that would translate into an increase in sexual arousal. As the data indicate, deviant sexual arousal as measured by penile circumference changes increased during the relaxation phase but dropped during covert sensitization. Subjective reports of arousal, however, actually dropped considerably during relaxation but rose during covert sensitization. There patients said they were much better during the relaxation phase and where ready to stop treatment. At no time did anyone say he was worse despite the fact that deviant arousal was increasing. Conversely, three patients said they were getting worse during covert sensitization although their deviant arousal was dropping daily. These data provide another example of splits amount the various response systems comprising sexual behaviour and the seeming ease with which these systems can be made to diverge. Yet another situation that may produce marked splits in response systems is the presence of strong legal contingencies. If certain sexual arousal patterns or behaviours will result in imprisonment or other legal sanctions, report of them will obviously not occur.

Contrived situations: The function of behavioural assessment in an ideal world would be the direct and continuous measurement of the three response systems comprising the behavioural problem in the setting where the behaviour presents a problem. Usually the setting is home, work, school, or social situations, or perhaps all these. Whatever the setting or combination of settings, it hasbecome known as the natural environment. Any procedure other than direct and continuous assessment of behaviour in the natural environment is second and continuous assessment of behaviour in the natural environment is second best. Yet in applied work this principle is constantly compromised for practical or ethical reasons. Thus clinicians cannot or will not measure practical or ethical reasons. Thus clinicians cannot or will not measure behaviour in the natural environment if it occurs in settings remote from he therapeutic setting, nor will they measure behaviour such as aggressive behaviour that occurs at very low frequencies. For ethical reasons clinicians also will not observe some behaviours such as sexual interactions in the natural environment beyond the very beginnings of this chain of behaviour (e.g., initial social approaches). To overcome these problems, contrived situations are devised to observe these behaviours at higher frequencies or in more convenient locations. In some cases the behaviours cannot be conveniently produced even in contrived situations. When this happens, as in the case of sexual behaviour, clinicians move back down the behavioural chain and measure sexual arousal, presumably an earlier component in the chain of sexual behaviour.

These are all necessary and helpful procedures,

but it is easy to lose sight of the fact that these measures are only as good as their relationship to the behaviour as it occurs in the natural environment. If these measures predict the occurrence or frequency of behaviour in the natural environment, then they are useful. If not, they are useless. Nevertheless, although one may read journals or listen to presentations on therapeutic intervention in clean experimental designs that demonstrate highly effective therapeutic procedures, one seldom questions the relationship of the analogue measures so commonly used in these clinical trials to behaviour in the natural environment. This observation is particularly applicable to studies of sexual behaviour.

A model of sexual behaviour: Early in the chapter we noted that sexual behaviour is more complex that the labels making up our well-known diagnostic categories would indicate. Glibly referring to certain behavioural patterns as "pedophilic" or "dysfunctional" may be useful from a descriptive point of view, but it vastly oversimplifies the components of sexual behaviour elucidated by recent research. First outlined in 1974, these components cut across all sexual problems. This chapter is organized around a description of procedures used to assess the various components of sexual behaviour. In the beginning of the chapter it was noted that there are three major components of sexual behaviour-sexual arousal, heterosexual social skills (hereafter referred to as heterosocial skills), and gender role deviations. Sexual problems may be biochemically or genetically based and there are sophisticated procedures for assessing these biochemical and genetic factors. However, it would not be appropriate to consider them in a chapter on behavioural assessment. Nevertheless the behavioural assessment strategies described in the next section are frequently used as auxiliary measures in the assessment of biochemically and genetically based sexual disorders.

Sexual arousal behaviour: The genital aspects of sexual behaviour have received the most attention over the years in studies of sexual problems, and thus assessment procedures utilizing the genitals are the most advanced. The genital component of sexual behaviour involves a chain of events beginning with the early aspects of sexual arousal through sexual contact of some kind and eventually orgasm. If two or more patterns of sexual arousal and/or behaviour are present, they may or may not be related to one another in terms of frequency or strength. For instance, some patients may have frequent heterosexual arousal and behaviour with a spouse and still often engage in alternative forms of sexual behaviour. The "true" bisexual and some fetishistic patients are included in this group. However, deviant sexual arousal is often accompanied by diminished heterosexual arousal. Diminished hetero-sexual arousal and behaviour do not, of course, necessarily imply the existence of alternative patterns of arousal.

Heterosocial skills: Most cultures have developed elaborate social patterns of behaviour surrounding the genital aspects of sexual behaviour. In our culture many patients may have adequate arousal patterns as well as the necessary behavioural repertoire to engage in the genital aspects of sex. However, these patients may be unable to engage in the type of heterosocial behaviours necessary for meeting, dating, and relating to desired persons. Similarly, many patients have adequate social skills but lack the necessary arousal patterns to engage in sexual behaviour.

Deviations in gender role: A percentage of patients, particularly those with certain patterns of deviant arousal, may have some degree of deviation in gender role. Behaviours appropriate to the opposite sex are present and some,e preference for the role of the opposite sex is verbalized. This is most common in homosexual or transvestite arousal patterns. When opposite sex behaviour is completely adopted and the patient consistently thinks, feels, and behaves in the opposite sex role this mistaken gender identity is called *transsexualism*. Such clients usually request surgery to reassign their sex.

Schema for the assessment of sexual behaviour: To summarize, there are three major components of sexual deviation. Each of these components may be assessed in either the natural environment or in contrived situations. Because each component of sexual behaviour can potentially be assessed in each of the three response systems) i.e., self-report, behavioural, physiological) and because these three response systems are relevant to both contrived and naturalistic settings, it is possible to construct a three-by-two grid along these dimensions that results in 18 cells. The remainder of this chapter will review current assessment procedures. Each of the behavioural assessment procedures described will fit into one of the cells of the schema.

Developmental models of human conduct are useful in showing how the numerous elements of a multifactor model interact across the lifespan. They help avoid debates about nature an nurture by clarifying how both biological and environmental factors influence behaviour at each phase of life.

The sexual reflexes function from the first days of life: Soon after birth, many boys have penile erections; and some girls, vaginal lubrication and clitoral tumescence. Even before birth, ultrasound studies suggest that erections may occur in male fetuses.

In the first year of life, many babies show the simplest forms of masturbation. Early in infancy, babies explore their environments and their own bodies, touching and looking at many parts of the anatomy with as much interest as they show for the world around them. Out of simple curiosity, they touch their arms, legs, and other parts, and discover their genitals in this process. Touch to the genitals elicits the sexual response, along with pleasurable feelings that reward genital self-stimulation. There are documented cases of babies learning to masturbate to orgasm before 1 year of age (though boys do not ejaculate any fluid before puberty). There is, however, considerable variation among children in early sexual self-stimulation, depending largely on their parent's response to the activity. Some parents punish and suppress early sexual behaviour; whereas others are more accepting. Children who are punished for genital exploration may not learn to touch their genitals. Punishment may in fact condition inhibitions and fears about self-touching.

Sometimes children are inquisitive to learn what other children's bodies look like. Since children's play is not always monitored closely by adults, sexual exploration can lead in many possible directions. Often it leads to nothing more than one child's simply looking at and brienfly touching the other child's body, but other outcomes are possible. A 9-year-old brother and his younger sister may innocently engage in mutual sexual exploration and discover that sexual play is pleasurable. In rare cases, after weeks of repeated sex play, they may discover intercourse, without knowing that adults would disapprove. Only later may the children discover that these activities are called "incest" and deemed unacceptable in the larger society.

In culture where people sleep together in a common room or hut, children may see their parents making love and later imitate coital activities during play with other children. There is a great deal of variability among children. There is a great deal of variability among cultures in childhood sexuality; and in societies where parents do not inhibit their children, sexual exploration and play continue throughout childhood: There is no biological determined "latency period" for sexuality.

In homes where early childhood sexual exploration is punished and little sexual information is given to the child, children can grow up with little knowledge and considerable guilt about touching their sexual organs or masturbating. Small degrees of such inhibition may not have long-lasting effects on the person's sexuality; but high levels of guilt and sexual ignorance can make it difficult for a person to develop a happy, uninhibited sexual life in subsequent years. Children who have negative socialization about sex often develop erotophobia, which is a fear of phobia of sexuality and sexual cues, leading to negative attitudes about sex. In contrast, a positive sexual socialization tends to lead to erotophilia, positive attitudes about sexuality and sexual cues.

In most societies, including ours, there is a double standard that imposes more sexual inhibitions, guilt, and erotophobia on girls than on boys. Parents are more likely to disapprove of masturbation for girls than boys. Girls are given fewer names for their genitals and are less likely to know the correct names than are boys, and few girls are told they have a clitoris. As a result, girls are less likely to masturbate or talk about their genitals than are boys.

Early Adolescence: Puberty usually begins between ages 9 and 13 in girls and 10 and 14 in boys. Most girls begin to menstruate between 11 to 14. Boys usually begin to be able to ejaculate at 11 to 12. The hormonal changes of puberty make the genitals more sensitive and more responsive. Adolescents—especially males—begin to experience spontaneous sexual arousal during the daytime and at night—in the form of noturnal sexual arousal, erections, and orgasms. As a result teenagers typically become increasingly interested in sexuality—unless they have been made to feel very guilty or inhibited about sex.

Boys typically develop sexual interests earlier and more intensely than girls. This is due to both biological and social factors. For biological reasons, boys usually begin to notice sexual arousal—such as spontaneous penile erections—2 or 3 years earlier than girls notice their first sexual arousal. Boys have more penile erections and orgasms—both while awake and sleeping—than girls have noticeable sexual arousal and orgasms. Boys are more likely than girls to be aware of their spontaneous sexual arousal and find it intense. Nocturnal erections occur during dream sleep and boys often wake in the morning with erections, which can help them discover the heightened level of pleasure that comes from masturbation after the onset of puberty. Also, boys have more nocturnal orgasms—or wet dreams—than do girls, and these are often coupled with sexual imagery that promote the development of sexual fantasies. As a result, the sexologist John Money calls wet dreams "nature's own pornography show"—just one more reason why boys tend to develop more erotic turn-ons and sexual fantasies than girls do.

There are exceptions to these generalization. Erotophobic boys may deny their emerging sexuality, and erotophilic girls may actively explore their sexuality, even though they experience fewer biological impulses to aid them than boys do. However, most boys feel sexual arousal and interest much more often each day than most girls do.

Boys are much more likely than girls to learn to masturbate to orgasm during the adolescent years. This is due, in parts, to the more frequent occurrences of spontaneous sexual arousal and orgasm in boys and the double standard that imposes less punishment and social inhibitions on boys than girls. In our culture, many boys also experience peer pressure to experiment with sexuality, gain sexual knowledge, and become "sexperts". Talk in the male peer group often turns to sex, and many boys feel pressure from their peer to lose their virginity and prove their manhood. Success is greeted with social approval, which rewards even more interest in sex.

Girls, in contrast, tend to experience a more

cautious socialization about sex. Yes, there is talk about sex in their peer groups, what it feels like and who is doing it. There is a great deal of variation among girls' peer groups, but these groups are more likely to pass on messages of caution about sex than are boys' peer groups. Girls learn that their more sexually active peers are called "sluts," or worse, and fear of social disparagement can make many girls reluctant to earn that label. Girls' peers may share frightening stories about girls who were taken advantage of by boys, stories of unwanted pregnancies and the subsequent problems, stories showing that STDs create many more complications for females than for males. In addition, girls may continue to hear words of caution from their parents.

Boys tend to want sex more than girls and to push more for it, while girls are more likely to play the gate-keeper role, wanting to know if he really cares about her before proceeding all the way to sexual intercourse. Hence, many girls and boys go through a period of petting or "fooling around" before engaging in sexual relations. Because physical touch to the skin, lips, and other body parts are all pleasurable, it is not surprising that couples enjoy the sensations of touching, fondling, kissing, and hugging. In such close interactions, pressure and touch to the genital areas are quite likely, which can heighten sexual arousal.

Erotic petting may be inhibited in societies that make young people feel guilty about premarital sex; or it can be facilitated in societies that inundate their youth with movies, videos, and stories of people doing sexual activities. Societal messages also influence the next step of sexual exploration: Societies with clear messages that premarital sex will be strongly punished may suppress further sexual exploration until marriage (or at least engagement); but such prohibitions are not very strong in most Western societies.

Premarital Sex: Many cultures have strict rules against premarital sex. Since most people throughout history have not had effective means of birth control, premarital sexual activity often led to pregnancy; and young unmarried mothers usually could not find marriage partners. Males often did not want to marry a pregnant woman or a woman or a woman with a child—unless it was theirs—because they did not want to devote their child-rearing efforts to raising someone else's children. In such cultures, virginity is very important; and a man may give a woman back to her family if she is found (or suspected) not to be a virgin at marriage. Naturally, there is much variation among cultures, and some societies allow a certain amount of premarital sex, perhaps with a fiance just before marriage.

Since the advent of the sexual revolution, many modern Western nations have experiences significant increases in premarital sexuality, this being due to the development of increasingly effective forms of birth control, the decreasing influence of rigid religious codes, and increased secular culture showing sexy images in videos, TV, and movies. In the United States, increasing premarital sex has led to an increasing amount of teenage pregnancy and teenage abortion, in part because many parents and teachers have been reluctant to provide good birth control information to teenagers. Even though a majority of American parents want sex education in the schools, a vociferous minority tends to block it in many schools. In Western Europe and Canada, where rates of teenage premarital sexual activity are similar to those in the United States, the teen pregnancy and abortion rates are considerably lower. For example, the pregnancy rate among 15 to 19 year olds is 96 per 1000 in the United States, compare to 35 per 1000 in Sweden and 14 per 1000 in the Netherlands. In modern Western European countries, teenagers are given better sexual education and better access to birth control services than in the United States. Also traditional religious influence is less powerful/influential in Europe.

While the prevalence of premarital sexual intercourse has gradually increased, the age of onset has gradually declined. For example, Alfred Kinsey, a pioneer sex researcher, found that half of the women he interviewed some 40 years ago had intercourse before marriage; but Morton Hunt found that 81% of 18- to 24-year-old married women had done so in the early 1970s. In 1971, only 46% of unmarried 19-year-old women had engaged in intercourse; but this percentage increased to 55% in 1976 and 69% in 1979. This trend for increasing early sexuality is believed to have leveled off in the 1980s. In 1990, 54% of high school students grades 9 to 12 have had sexual intercourse.

Most parents do not tell their children or adolescents many details about the scripts for sexual intercourse, and many signal a reluctance or unwillingness to talk about premarital sex. As a result, many teens turn to their peers and the media for this information. These multiple and different sources often provide confusing or inaccurate information, with jumbled and often contradictory messages about the events surrounding first sex. Because it can be difficult to tell which of the countless different scripts presented by the media and peers is the best, adolescents often experiment with numerous lines and scripts, combining elements from various ones, not knowing which ones will work best for them until they have tried many. The less accurate information they have, the more likely are to make mistakes. Because many of the scripts used on TV and in movies do not work well in everyday life, adolescence can involve much frustrating experimentation and embarrassment. (The more accurate information that teens receive from parents, sex educators, and books, the more likely they are to be well prepared for adolescent sexual exploration and first intercourse.)

In a study of girls' experience around the time they have their first sex, Sharon Thompson found that many girls worried about a boy's putting a "big thing in small hole." Many did not know the ways that boys are likely to approach them for first sex and are surprised by the rapidity with which first sex occurred. Some were taken advantage of because they did not have realistic expectations and scripts for dealing with the boys. Those girls who were least likely to be abused or taken advantage of during their early sexual activities had mothers who talked honestly with them about the sexual scripts needed for good experiences with sex. First intercourse is usually less problematic for boys than girls. Typically, boys have orgasm and like losing their virginity. Girls are less likely to orgasm and less happy about their loss of virginity. However, after a year or two of sexual experience, many females and males begin to learn which scripts work best, how to have better sex, and how to avoid some of the problems related to sex—such as pregnancy, sexually transmitted disease (STDs) and abusive partners.

Although some parents may believe that a guilt-inducing sex socialization will keep their child from experimenting with premarital sex, the erotophobia they condition in their children can create serious problems. Erotophobic teens often feel so guilty about sex that they avoid sex education information and do not learn effective means of birth control. This can leave them vulnerable to sexual accidents if their erotophobia is overcome by curiosity about sex or pressure from another person to experiment with sex. Although students with high sex guilt may begin sex as early as students with low sex guilt, they wait about a year longer than those with low sex guilt before using contraception. Erotophobic people can become pregnant and contract sexually transmitted diseases as easily as other people; and their lack of knowledge about sex puts them at a greater risk of such mishaps, since they have not planned ahead for sex and have limited knowledge about ways to avoid the problems.

Since AIDS has become a serious health problem, considerable efforts has been directed at teaching adolescents safer practices—such as the use of condoms and avoiding anal sex. Although some teens are following this advice, many teens are not using condoms for safer sex. In 1991, 46% of high school students reported using condoms during their last sexual intercourse. Since one-fifth of all people with AIDS contracted the virus as teens, there is room for improvement in education and honest communication with teens about sex.

Cohabitation: Although cohabitation is less common in the United States than in France or Sweden, increasing numbers of people are living with a partner without being married. In the United States, approximately 4% of unmarried adults are cohabiting, in contrast to 1% in 1960.

In the early 1950s, the typical age of marriage was about 20 years in women and 22.5 in men. Today it is about 24 in women and 26 in men. Since teens are also beginning sex at earlier ages than in the 1950s, it is clear that many young people are spending more years of their lives as sexually active but unmarried than was true before the sexual revolution. Some individuals have 2 to 5 years before they enter a relationship that will lead to marriage; for others it may be 10 years or more. Those who post-pone marriage are more likely to cohabit than those who do not.

People who cohabit tend to be more liberal, and less religious, and more critical of marriage as an institution than people who do not cohabit. Although cohabitation is becoming increasingly routine before marriage, there is no evidence that it helps people make better choices of marital partners. Most cohabiting unions do not lead to marriage, dissolving relatively quickly. Also, cohabitors are more likely to divorce than people who do not cohabit, perhaps because they are more critical of marriage both before and after the wedding.

Marriage: In their 20s and 30s, married couples typically engage in coitus two or three times a week. Erotophiles often seek out ways to expand their sexual lives, add new activities and keep their erotic love strong. Many erotophobes expected that sex would be good once it was legitimated by marriage; but even after marriage, many erotophobes continue to feel that sex is "dirty," "sinful," or "base"; and these feelings can interfere with the enjoyment of intimate sexual relations for years or all through life.

The frequency of intercourse usually declines as people age. Many married people report that sexual relations are most fulfilling in the first year after marriage and that the quality of their sexual experience declines thereafter. People also report a decline in communication, listening, respect, and romantic love after marriage. These changes are not biologically determined or inevitable; but they do indicate that many people do not devote much attention to making their marriages successful. They also suggest that many people do not have the time, effort, or skill to solve their marital and sexual problems and/or that the multiple other demands of adult life—jobs, careers, children, socializing—are so demanding or rewarding that their marriages become neglected.

Heterosexual couples commonly engage in noncoital sex play before penile-vaginal intercouse, Foreplay typically lasts some 5 to 15 minutes, though the time varies from couple to couple and from time to time for any given couple. Various stimulative techniques are used in foreplay, including touching, caressing, and kissing of the genitals, breasts, lips, and other body parts. Couples use a variety of positions for engaging in intercourse, which usually lasts approximately 10 minutes. While the male-on-top, face-to-face position is very common, couples are increasingly using the female-on-top position. Side-by-side positions and combinations of female superior and side-by-side positions are also used. Rearentry positions are less commonly explored.

Many couples engage in oral-genital stimulation. Hunt's research found that 90% of people married less than 25 years had engaged in oral sex during the preceding year. Anal intercourse is not a common practice for most couples. Hunt's data indicate that for married people between 18 and 25, approximately 50% of men and 25% of women had engaged in anal intercourse on at least one occasion. A 1991 study of men ages 20-39 found that 20% had engaged in anal intercourse, 75% had performed oral sex, and 79% had received it. Gay and lesbian couples use manual and oral stimulation of the genitals, breasts, and anus, along with caressing, kissing, and body rubbing for sexual arousal. Since the advent of AIDS, many gay males have reduced their use of anal sex, since it is one of the activities most likely to transmit HIV (the virus that causes AIDS).

Although females tend to be less interested in sex than males in the teens and 20s, female sexual interest tends to increase in 20s, 30s, and 40s. Many of the inhibitions that girls learned while young are gradually overcome. As women learn how to avoid irresponsible partners, unwanted pregnancies, and STDs, they learn how to avoid some of the problems that had cuased them to worry about sex earlier. Also, many learn how to have orgasms more easily, making sex more exciting and fulfilling. Many overcome guilt and other inhibitions as supportive sexual partners, the legitimacy of marriage, and access to more reliable information about sex counteract earlier fears and myths (ignorance). These factors have led many to the generalization that male sex drive peaks at 20 while females peak in their 30s or 40s. This generalization is somewhat misleading, since (1) many males have very strong sexual interests all through young and middle adulthood, and some even longer, and (2) increasing numbers of young women have fewer sexual inhibitions or are overcoming their sexual inhibitions at an earlier age than their mothers did. Modern books, courses, and workshops on sexuality help them do this.

People in their teens and 20s often explore novel sexual positions and activities, but married couples often settle into a few favorite positions after they have explored a range of possibilities and discovered the ones they like the best. This can eventually lead to boredom with sex. If married couples report that they are losing interest in sex because it has become too routine, sexual therapists and marriage counselors sometimes give couples books that show multiple sexual positions and encourage them to try novel ones.

Extramarital sex: Although marriage vows require faithfulness, studies reveal that a considerable number of people break the traditional marital contract. Hunt's survey in the 1970s found that 50% of married men and 20% of married women had at least one extramarital relationship by the age of 45. However, the rates for younger women were similar of those of men. Other more recent surveys of magazine readers indicate higher rates of extramarital sex. For example, a Cosmopolitan survey found that 60% of the women and 75% of men had extramarital sexual experience. There is historical and cross-cultural evidence that extramarital sex has been common at other times and in other societies. Although most individuals attempt to keep their extramarital affairs secret, they do not always succeed; and the discovery that there has been extramarital sex can be very damaging to the quality of a marriage, undermining trust and sometimes leading to divorce.

Some people, most notably Nena and George O'Neil in the book *Open Marriage,* recognize that secret affairs are common yet potentially deleterious to marriage and advocate "open marriage" as an alternative. Built on the assumption that most people want both a committed relationship and freedom, open marriage is designed to allow a couple to see other people and decide if this should include sexual relations or not. There are too few studies on open marriage to know how common it is. One study found that in 15% of marriages, both partners had agreed that extramarital sex was acceptable under certain circumstances.

About 50% of marriages end in divorce in the United States, though there has been a gradual decline in divorce since its peak in 1981. For many couples, marital happiness is the highest in the first year of marriage. As incompatibilities and fights begin to detract from the feelings of love, many couples cease to feel the passion and commitment needed to keep a relationship together. The peak in divorce occurs at 1.5 years after marriage. Many married people stop trying as hard at making their relationship work, and many experience a decline in marital happiness, sexual pleasure, and love. This need not occur if people continue to value their relationship and put time and effort into it. Unfortunately, the numerous obligations of adulhood—job, parenthood, maintaining a home—can take so many hours a week that many adults simply do not have the time to devote to their relationship. Thus, one study found that "difficulty in communication" was the most common reason given for divorce. Other reasons were unhappiness and incompatibility. Also, the birth of the first child is one of the greatest stresses on a relationship, and the sooner the child comes after marriage, the greater the chances of divorce. Waiting a couple of years before beginning a family allows a couple to solve many of their interpersonal problems and establish a stable relationship before adding the complexities of childrearing. Counselors, marriage workshops, and books can help, too.

Few topics regarding human behaviour hold as much interest and as much pathos as that of deviations and dysfunctions in human sexuality. What constitutes deviations and dysfunctions, however, are heavily dependent on contemporary cultural attitudes and values and these are often blind to the past history of sexuality in the culture.

We know, for example, that sexuality was represented in the rock art of the earliest human cultures. Paleolithic (30,000 to 10,000 B.C.) rock art, for example, is replete with both human and animal fertility symbols that were thought to endow the represented forms with abundant offspring. The Egyptians (3000 B.C.) are thought to have added power to the concept of fertility as represented in their symbols. In Western culture, our sexual values came mostly from the Judeao—Christian traditions. The Judaic tradition emphasized reproductive sexual behaviour without guilt. The core concern was to protect the integrity of marriage with all other considerations of secondary value. Strict laws of adultery were applied to women but the husband was instructed only to "not covet your neighbour's wife...," otherwise sex outside the marriage was tolerated. While the Jews were nomadic and their values emphasized family and procreation, sexual values for the Greeks emanated from their more settled agricultural lifestyle. Here family was still central but the Greeks allowed far more freedom of sexual expression in varied forms. For example, bisexuality was common among Greek males. Since beauty was the primary value or attraction, sexual behaviour and arousal could arise in response to both boys and young or mature women of beauty. With the rise of Christianity more ascetic beliefs began to emerge. In general, sex had a procreative function, not the pleasure role noted with the Greeks and Hebrews. By the 18th century, religious views of life shifted from emphasis on eternal life in heaven to attaining happiness on earth and romantic love was valued. Sexual "deviations" started to become cultural issues with particular emphasis on homosexuality and masturbation. As venereal diseases became widespread, cultural values shifted to the physician as the arbiter of sexual morality, and to the repression of sexual behaviour, particularly that of males. In the 20th century sexual notions are clearly shifting towards a continuum of behaviours. Modern sexologists not only have described the physiological, emotional, and psychological aspects of sexual behaviour but have also highlighted the various forms of sexual behaviour that exist whether in overt or covert forms.

This article deals with the full range of human sexual thoughts, feelings, and actions that are generally regarded as abnormal, deviant, or disordered. Our focus will be on these extremes but it should be noted that "deviant" and "disordered" are concepts that rest upon the assumption of a medical, disease, or psychiatric model of behaviour that dichotomizes human actions into two qualitatively separate categories of "normal" and "abnormal." Some sexologists, on the other hand, view these sexual behaviour variations not as diseases to be cured but as atypical expressions representing quantitative rather than qualitative differences. To them, sexual behaviour falls on a broad continuum with the extremes being vunerable to labels like "disordered" and "abnormal." Here we are dealing with difference in intensity and narrowness of behaviour rather than qualitatively different behaviours. We can see this, for example, in the husband who might be aroused by his wife wearing lingerie versus the fetish individual who can only become sexually aroused by lingerie. Furthermore, the demarcation between abnormal and normal categories is not fixed or absolute. Rather, it consists of an ever changeable subjective value judgment derived from psychiatric, cultural, and political forces. For example, masturbation, once considered a sin then a disease, is now acceptable and understood. Likewise, homosexuality was actually removed from the psychiatric nomenclature due to political pressures and changes in culture norms. These are examples of the changeable nature of categorization and labeling and the subjective social value judgments they represent.

Our discussion will follow closely the psychiatric nomenclature and diagnostic categories since these represent our current values regarding human sexuality and the types of behaviours that are considered unacceptable in mainstream society.

We will use the terms or labels often used in psychiatry and law to denote these patterns. Although it is not a psychiatric disorder, we will discuss homosexuality since it is a form of sexual behaviour that has socio-cultural historical relevance and is still a controversial topic among some peoples. We will also discuss rape, gender identity disorders, and sexual addictions which are listed in the psychiatric diagnostic system but not under sexual disorders.

The behavioural area of sexual dysfunctions is not discussed since it usually represents inhibitions in sexual drive or performance and is not as comprehensive a manifestation of one's being as are the problems and stresses characteristic of sexual disorders. Finally, we will briefly discuss the topic of rape, emphasizing its aggressive and violent nature rather than sexual nature.

Our starting place in discussing sexual disorders is to focus on the notion of "sexual identity." A person's sexual identity can be seen as an interrelationship among the three basic elements of human sexual behaviour, namely, biological sexual characteristics, gender identity, and sexual orientation. In the diagram below you can see that sexual identity is formed from the interaction between biological sex characteristics (such as male and female sex organs, hormones, etc.), gender identity (or one's identification with or feeling of feminity or masculinity), and sexual orientation (homo-, bi-, hetero-sexual, or other objects of stimulation as found, for example, in the paraphilas). In examining the gender identity disorders we will be discussing biological sex and gender identity. On the other hand, when we discuss the paraphilias, we will be focusing in part upon sexual orientation.

Gender identity disorders: A person with gender identity disorder (GID) experiences a confusion or mismatch between biological sexual characteristics and their culturally assigned gender identity. The identity problem is psychological in nature rather than a biological ambiguity. Biologically, they are dimorphic (male vs female) in terms of chromosomal, gonadal, gential development, and hormonal levels. The ambiguity exists in terms of the individual's identification with culturally defined traits that constitute being a woman or man, i.e., the degree of femininity or masculinity the person exhibits through thoughts, feelings, and their actions. Not all people are comfortable with what they feel is their true sense of being a woman or man and their biological sex. The amount of disturbance can range from a mild sense of inappropriateness, to feeling like a woman trapped in a male's body, and vice versa.

GID should not be confused with transvestitism, homosexuality, and hermaphroditism. Transvestites, as we will see later in more detail, cross-dress for fetishistic pleasure, and, with few exceptions, rarely find an incongruity between their sex and gender. A person who is emotionally and sexually attracted to a member of their same sex is, likewise, not inherently disturbed in regards to their gender identity. Finally, the hermaphrodite has to some degree the sexual organs for both sexes. Since this confusion stems from being biologically intersexed, the hermaphrodite's dilemma is not considered a psychological disorder. Once again, those with GID are unambiguously biologically formed in one sex, and their confusion is at the emotional and psychological levels. GIDs are conceptually divided into three categories : GID of childhood, GID of adolescence and adulthood (not transsexual), and trans-sexualism.

Gender Identity Disorder of Childhood: GID of childhood is reserved for prepubescent children and is relatively uncommon. The sex ratio for the population in general is unknown, yet through clinical work it appears that there are many more boys than girls diagnosed with this condition. Generally, the age of onset for both sexes is age 4; however, in some cases it may appear as early as age 2. The majority of children will return to their expected gender roles by puberty, while the remaining minority will continue experiencing what is called "gender dysphoria" or role confusion. Reliable predictions of adult pathology, based upon nontypial childhood behaviour have proved elusive. The primary symptoms needed to make a diagnosis are : (1) a persistent and severe discomfort regarding her or his own biological sex, and (2) a belief that they are, or desire to be, of the opposite sex. Such feelings and behaviours are chronic and problematic, thereby transcending any normal variation of stereotypical gender roles, such as being a "tomboy" or a "sissy."

A female with this disorder exhibits intense feelings of frustration at being a girl with a corresponding desire to become a boy, or, in some case, they may even believe that they are of the opposite gender already. They often seek male peers and are repulsed by traditional feminine toys, games, etc., preferring instead the masculine equivalents. Lastly, there is an intense disgust toward and rejection of their anatomy, often illustrated by beliefs that they will grow a penis or not go through normal female pubescent body changes. The overall pattern with males is identical to the female description except that the specifics are reverse. For example, GID boys typically show severe distress at being a boy, they engage in cross-dressing, and prefer female toys, peers, and so on. They are repulsed by their genitalia, often wishing that it would disappear or that they would grow up and become a woman.

A major difference between the two sexes is found in the fact that many more boys than girls are treated for this condition. It is thought that differential socialization patterns may account for the discrepancy in prevalence rates. For example, boys are more often subjected to rigid parental expectations and therefore any nontypial gender behaviour is often more apparent. Boys also tend to display more signs of secondary pathology, e.g., depression, anxiety, and withdrawal, perhaps due to harsher social consequences from peers for their feminine-like behaviour. On the other hand, females who cross the gender lines ("tomboys") tend to be more readily accepted than "sissies," or boys who violate gender expectations.

Gender identity disorder of adolescence or adulthood (Nontrassexual): A person with this condition must have reached puberty, exhibit reoccurring discomfort with their biological sex, and habitually cross-dress. Motivation for wearing the apparel of the opposite sex is for emulation purposes, not for fetishistic pleasure. They are psychologically identified with the opposite sex and exhibit intermittent to constant cross-dressing. Despite the person's sense of discomfort, they usually have no preoccupations with changing their sex to match their gender identity.

Some researchers theorize that GIDs should be conceptualized on a continuum rather than as separate diagnostic categories. Accordingly, they might prefer the term transgenderism, which can be seen as an intermediate stage between the two extremes of GID of childhood and secondary transsexualism, i.e., someone who after a period of time decides to make a sex change. The transgenderist is someone who is living permanently in the role of the opposite sex but does not have the desire for a complete sex change. Essentially, their change is in gender, not in sexual biological characteristics.

Transsexualism: The transsexual condition can be distinguished from other GIDs essentially because of a life-long sense of gender incongruence or inappropriateness and a persistent preoccupation or obsessive quest for sex realignment or "reassignment" surgery. This preoccupation for sex change surgery must be present for a least 2 years to be diagnosed transsexualism. As you can see, we are now at the more extreme end of the GID continuum.

Some theorists have attempted to distinguish between primary and secondary transsexualism, with the former evidencing a history of gender dysphoria since childhood while the latter may be long-term cross-dressers or transgenderists but they seek reassignment surgery later in life usually after experiencing a traumatic stressor.

Secondary pathology for transsexuals is common and most often includes anxiety and depression. For those who are driven to change their sex, the difficulty in getting the funds to pay for surgery can result in self-mutilation and even suicide. In a culture that defines their dilemma as pathological and abnormal, transsexuals have many stories to relate about the pain and suffering they experience. This brief glimpse into the recollection of a girl "trapped" in a male body should partially convey their struggle for recognition as legitimate human beings:

> ... I wanted above all to walk down the hall at school and be looked at and respected as were the normal girals, yes, normal girls; for I was a girl with all my heart, but I was not a normal girl. I was a freak of a girl, one who had to look like a boy.

It is generally believed that transsexualism is present in about 1 out of 30,000 males and 1 out of every 100,000 females. More males seek out treatment than females, with ratios as high as 8 to 1. In the United States alone, it is estimated that there are between six and ten thousand postoperative transsexuals, i.e., people who have had sex change operations.

Etiology of gender identity disorders: As the current body of knowledge now stands, the causal roots of GID remain undiscovered. The various approaches that attempt to explain this particular disorder can be broken down into the biological/ medical, psychodynamic, and developmental/ learning models. The first approach purposes genetic, hormonal, neurological, and chromosomal abnormalities as a causal factor. Despite a few leads, such as the effects of prenatal hormones on gender behaviour, there is meager amount of data to support the notion of biology as a sole or even major influence. The psychodynamic model emphasizes early childhood and personality development. Causal roles are attributed to difficulty with mother-child relations and the failure to psychologically identify with the parent of the opposite sex. Again, this is not a universal or even major phenomenon. Furthermore, it is very difficult to tease out what is the chicken and what is the egg. In other words, do parents shape children's behaviour or does the child's behaviour shape the parents' difficulty with the relationship? Finally, the importance of socialization processes and the acquisition of atypical childhood behaviours via modeling or conditioning represents the learning and development point of view. Unfortunately, contrary to both the psychodynamic and learning models, there is very little indication that the family environment has any serious effect in the development of gender identity disorders for substantial numbers of cases. For example, in a study by R. Green, of 16 children who were raised by transsexuals all were found to have heterosexual orientation with no disturbance in their gender identity.

Treatment approaches to gender identity disorders: The general consensus is that many or all behavioural and psychodynamic treatments for GID are ineffective. Behavioural therapies have produced a few "success" in strongly motivated clients, but even then some of the behavioural modification techniques used have raise disturbing moral questions. For example, reports of behaviour therapies describe asking children to overemphasize the gender identity differences so as to produce aversive social reactions which, presumably, would diminish these opposite-sex behaviours and attitudes. In contrast, psychodynamic treatments aim at resolving childhood conflicts in the hope of producing acceptance of one's sex and the corresponding gender identity. After many case histories and grueling therapeutic hours, personality reorganization approaches have almost always ended in total failure. Both approaches subject children to personal pain in addition to the feelings of failure they must experience in therapies that are ineffective.

For transsexuals, sex reassignment treatment (sex change surgery) has proven in a majority of cases to be successful in bringing happiness and relief. After a careful screening process, a qualified individual must undergo intensive counseling and instruction on matters of grooming, vocation, legal rights, voice training, and the proper use of stereotypical gender role mannerisms. Then they may begin hormonal therapy in order to produce the desired secondary sex characteristics, e.g., breasts in males facial/body hair modification, changes in body fat distribution, and some voice alteration. After living and working in one's new gender role for 1 to 2 years, only then can the candidate undergo genital reconstruction. The artificially constructed vagina is much more realistic in appearance and function than its male counterpart. While female genitalia is capable of lubrication and orgasm, the penis is less sensitive and lacks natural erectile capacities. Though limited in number and with sometimes inconclusive findings, some follow-up studies have indicated an 80 to 85% satisfaction rate for transsexual operations, with male-to-female transsexuals usually faring better than their counterparts. Dissatisfaction is usually the result of poor surgical techniques and personal and social instability that preceded surgery.

The paraphilias: The term paraphilia is derived from the notion of a deviation or separation (para-) from what most people are attracted to (-philia). Originally, these were called "perversions," but modern terminology generally describes then as "deviations" or, more recently, as "variations." The DSM-III-R describes these deviations as "...recurrent sexual urges and sexually arousing fantasies generally involving either (1) nonhuman objects, (2) to suffering or humiliation of oneself or one's partner (not merely simulated), or (3) children or nonconsenting persons." The diagnosis, however, is made only if the person has acted on there urges or is greatly disturbed or distressed about them. Paraphilic fantasy (such as sex with animals, arousal from undergarments, sado-masochistic thoughts, cross-dressing, or sex with children, etc.) as such is not sufficient to warrant clinical diagnosis. These preoccupations must be intense and recurrent, or undesired and disturbing to the individual, the preferred or exclusive forms of sexual gratification, or acted out overtly to be considered pathological. The paraphilias are usually multiple in nature rather than singular. They are almost exclusively confined to men with the exception of masochism, in which we see a significant number of females.

Current views of paraphilias have been heavily influenced by Freudian theory and analysis of sexual behaviour. Within the psychodynamic model, a healthy or natural sexual relationship consists of opposite sexed partners whose object is coitus (sexual gratification through intercourse). These deviation in sexual orientation involve the use of an object other than the opposite sex partner, such as one of the same sex (homosexual), children (pedophilia), close relative (incest), animals (zoophilia), inanimate objects (fetish), or even dead people (necrophilia), as sexual objects. Likewise, instead of seeking coitus, departures include watching others (voyeurism), exposing genitals (exhibitionism), infliction of pain (sadism), or suffering pain (masochism) as deviant aims. In the paraphilias, the erotic object has a role or characteristic that is more important than their personality and personal characteristics of the object and the aim is to enact the paraphilic fantasy.

Mainstream diagnostic systems have been strongly influenced by these two major departures from object and aim. Alternatively, others have argued that perhaps the impact on others should be used as the diagnostic criterion. Here, fetishes and transvestism, and perhaps gender identity disorders, would be excluded in that they usually have little or no direct negative impact on others. All this is brought to your attention to highlight the subjective and consequently changing nature of diagnosis and categorization. Basically, as with most other mental illness categories, we are dealing with social value judgments rather than specific "diseases" and as such cultural and political values and attitudes influence the diagnostic process.

Pedophilias: The pedophile (derived from the Greek for "child lover") sexually prefers children of either sex for erotic gratification. It is usually thought that perpetuators must be at least 10 years older than their victims, but this age difference may differ considerably depending on circumstances. Pedophilia is also called "child sexual abuse" and "child molestation." Child molestation is most often perpetrated by males and usually involves such actions as manipulation of the child's genitalia, stroking of the body, forcing the child to manipulate the adult's genitalia, and, to a lesser degree, intermission. Pedophilia is the most common form of paraphilias and involves the most vulnerable victims-children.

Heterosexual men are responsible for most sex abuse against girls. Two out of three sexually abused children, however, are girls. Conservative estimates are that 10% of females and 2% of males were sexually abused as children. There is no well—delineated personality for the pedophilic. However, the concept of the "dirty old man" as perpetuator is misguided in that most pedophiles are in their late 30s with only about 5% being aged men. If we had to generalize, we could say that pedophiles are generally immature developmentally even though they may have married and have children of their own. Second, we often see the behaviour under stress, i.e., during stressful life periods often accompanied by marital and sexual problems. Alcohol is consistently involved in pedophilic encounters. The majority of victims are relatives, neighbours, or acquaintances; and encounters, while usually brief, occur in series of extended contacts. Generally the younger the child, the more immature the perpetuator. Actual penetration and coitus occur in only 4% of cases. Interestingly, the vast majority (80%) of perpetuators have themselves been abused as children.

Incest: Incest is treated here as a subcategory of pedophilia. However, since pedophiles differ in age from their victim, incest may not necessarily meet the criteria. For example, the majority of incest cases seem to involve cousins and siblings who might be similar in age. Incest (from the Latin "impure") is a form of pedophilia involving close relatives, most commonly between cousins but parent-child or sibling-sibling incest is the most repugnant and most often the focus of treatment or criminal proceedings. Taboos against incest are present in all cultures, particularly against mother-son incest. Surveys among adults indicate that 14% of males reported having had sexual contact with a relative before adulthood (95% of which were heterosexual in nature) and 9% of females have had such contact. Most of these experiences were with cousins and essentially involved some form of "petting." Among a university sample, however, 10% of females reported incestuous relationships with their fathers (including stepfathers). Almost 90% of cases brought to court for incest involve father-daughter while only 5% are father-son incidents. Transgenerational incest seems to occur in about 10% of incest cases but probably has different dynamics than immediate parents and children or children and children.

The studies of incest have concluded that these events occur within seriously disturbed or dysfunctional families and that a code of silence develops in which these events are not spoken bout and often repressed by the victims. Furthermore, the parents in this unhappy marriage typically consists of a domineering, authoritative, and impulsive husband and a dependent and emotionally distant wife. The husbands often also abuse the wives as well as the children.

Incest is a criminal as well as psychological disorder. The experience of incest is traumatic and psychologically damaging to the children involved (and even to those who know about it). Criminal prosecution does not erase the trauma of incest. These deep psychological scars must eventually be addressed in order for the victim to heal and live a fully mature life.

Voyeurism: Voyeurs are also called "peepers" or "Peeping Toms." The psychiatric diagnostic system describes this condition as a recurrent, intense, and sexually oriented "act of observing unsuspecting people, usually strangers, who are either naked, in the process of disrobing, or engaging in sexual activity..." Looking (or "peeping") provides sexual arousal but no actual sexual contact with the observed person is sought. Orgasm, usually produced by masturbation, may occur during the voyeuristic activity, or later in response to the memory of what the person has witnessed. Often these people enjoy the fantasy of having a sexual experience with the observed person, but in reality this does not occur. In its severe form, peeping constitutes the exclusive form of sexual activity.

Lady Godiva's ride through the streets of Coventry to remit an oppressive tax was watched by no one from the town—out of respect and gratitude for her actions—with the exception of Tom the tailor, who peeped through the curtains and for this act went blind. The "Peeing Tom" of today does not go blind literally but they are almost always men. To be considered a paraphilia, there must be a recurrent and intense preoccupation with looking from hiding or secret places. Just looking at live nudes or pictures of nudes is not a paraphilia.

Voyeurs tend to be younger men (convicted age is 23.8 years), unmarried and with little or no alcohol, drug, or other mental illness problems.

While they tend to be a heterogeneous as a group, they do commonly have deficiencies in heterosexual relationships. As a matter of fact, it has been conjectured that the voyeuristic practices are a safe and protected way of avoiding a possible relationship with a woman.

Exhibitionism: The legal term for exhibitionism is "indecent exposure" because of the shock or offensive value of the act to others. Again, this is mainly a male disorder. Like other paraphilias, it involves repetition, intensity, and sexual urges or arousing fantasies of at least 6 months duration. For the exhibitionist or "flasher" gratification seems to come from the disgust, shock, fear, and surprise of the unsuspecting usually female victims. There is usually a compulsive, driven quality to this behaviour (as with most paraphilias) but they are also prone to be caught as they return to the same situation or place repeatedly. There is some evidence that at some level they may wish to be caught and that this consequence is deliberate and desired. The exhibitionists' behaviour has a distinctive hostile air to it and this, coupled with the fact that they often have serious sexual problems might suggest intense, perhaps unconscious, hostility exists toward women. As a group they tend to be younger (30s) with about 30% married, 30% divorced or separated, and 40% never married. They are often above average in intelligence and do not have more serious forms of mental illness.

Anxiety, which forms a part in all the paraphilias, is also apparent in exhibitionists both in terms of the excitement or anxiety associated with the act itself and with the desire for anxiety relief that results from the act. There is also evidence that exhibitionists are sexually aroused by stimuli that usually have little or no arousal potential for most people (such as seeing fully clothed women in normal activities) and thus may misread the motives and intentions of others (perhaps seeing them as sex crazed as they are). A fairly large percentage of women (between 45 and 50%) report having seen or had direct contact with a "flasher."

Fetishism: Fetishism involves sexual arousal from some inanimate or nonliving object. Exposure to the object or preference for the object is usually necessary to maintain erectile states. Common objects include shoes, sheer stockings, gloves, toilet articles, undergarments particularly underpants, and many tactilely stimulating substances (soft fetishes) such as fur, velvet, and silk garments, and smooth solid objects (hard fetishes) that can be rubbed and fondled such as shoes, leather objects, and so on.

In ancient cultures, fetishes were objects that had magical powers. For the fetishist the object itself is endowed with sexual power and the owner is of little or no interest. Panties, stockings, and garders may be alluring and channel excitment to the wearer but to the fetishist, the object itself is the allure and goal, not the user.

Almost any object can acquire fetish properties. One mechanism for acquisition is classical conditioning in which a neutral object comes to acquire arousal properties by association with sexual arousal and stimulation (i.e., masturbating with the object present). By this process, any stimulus, even body parts, can become a fetish object.

Orgasm may occur with the fetish alone or the fetish object may need to be present during intercourse in order to maintain stimulation toward orgasm. Again, poorly developed heterosexual relationships are found in fetishes as in other paraphilias. Here, however, there is usually a strong mother-son bond with the fetish individual. Fetishes usually develop during adolescence. They are seldom distraught enough by the behaviour to seek out psychotherapy and they are usually not overt or foolish enough to be arrested or detected.

Transvestism: The Latin trans meaning "across" and vestia meaning "dress" for the term for "cross-dressing" or "transvestism." As pointed out earlier, transsexuals often manifest cross-dressing as a first expression of opposite sex feelings. This behaviour, along with men who dress in "drag" to attract other men for sexual purposes, is not usually considered manifestations of transvestism. Likewise, female impersonators and actors who play female parts are not included under this diagnosis. To qualify as transvestism, there must be a compulsive desire to cross-dress and an intense frustration when the practice is interfered with. The transvestite is usually heterosexual in orientation, married, and otherwise masculine in appearance, demeanor, and sexual preference. The cross-dressing, while compulsive, is done in secret and does not lead to homosexuality or gender identity problems—although transvestites report feeling like a woman during the cross-dress episodes. Often wives will be overt or covert conspirators in the cross-dressing activities. Cross-dressers will often seek each other out for social occasions while made up as women.

The compulsion to cross-dress begins by adolescence, although most children who cross-dress will "grow out of it" by adulthood. Some male transvestites recall their parents forcing them to wear girls clothing as a form of humiliation and punishment. As an adult, however, the wearing of women's clothing usually has more significance than just sexual arousal or punishment. If affords the transvestite male an opportunity to escape from pressures and responsibilities. Some males only partially cross-dress, usually by covertly wearing female undergarments under their male clothing. Others are complete cross-dressers, who overtly carry out this practice either occasionally or, for some, all the time.

Sadomasochism (S-M): The term sadomasochism is derived from the family names of two historical characters. The first is the French nobleman Marquis de Sade, whose writing consisted of vivid accounts of pain inflicted on one partner in sexual encounters of various kinds. Sexual sadism is defined as the inflection of physical pain and/or personal humiliation and degradation on a sexual partner. While de Sade portrayed infliction of excruciating pain on individuals, most sadism involves mild to moderate pain. It is estimated that about 5% of men and 2% of women have obtained sexual pleasure by inflicting pain on a regular basis.

While sadists inflict pain on willing or nonconsenting partners, sexual masochists (from Leopold von Sacher-Masoch, a German novelist who described this behaviour in the late 19th century) enjoy suffering for erotic excitement as a preferred form of sexual activity. While sadists overwhelmingly tend to be men, masochists are more often females. The study of sadomasochism has only just begun. What little is known about these practices comes mainly from case studies, i.e., examination of S-M activities at centers for such activities or through paid dominance and submission sexual surrogates hired for these purposes.

Sadomasochistic activities center on use of dominance-aggression and submission in sexual activities. Terms that denote these activities abound such as bondage and domination (B-D), master-mistress, dominatrix, humiliation, restraints, whipping, leather/rubber, slave, bottom or submissive, and so on. Activities often involve elaborate interaction, sometimes with predetermined code words that will lead to the immediate release of a victim if desired and often use fetishistic trappings such as leather/rubber garments, chains, whips, shackles, harnesses, and other props. Rarely do sadomasochistic practices lead to physical injury, mutilation, or death. Victims, however, may be nonconsenting or willing and, not infrequently, paid sexual partners. The most frequent S-M activities are spanking, master-slave bondage, humiliation situations, oral-anal S-M contexts, whipping, and to a lesser degree, verbal abuse, enemas, torture, "golden showers" (urinating on someone), and use of toilet articles.

There is a well-defined S-M subculture that includes paraphernalia sex shops, stages for bondage scenes, magazines, prostitutes trained in S-M skills, and videos. Participants are predominantly heterosexual males with a greater concentration of bisexual female participants. Sadomasochistic activities are defined as paraphilisa if they are recurrent and intense. To just tie up a sexual partner occasionally is not S-M activity.

Miscellaneous Paraphilias: Sexual arousal can become conditioned to a wide variety of eliciting stimuli. In this section, we will describes some relatively uncommon paraphilias that involve usual and sometimes noxious objects of sexual arousal. The miscellaneous paraphilias described below not only occur rarely but are often not detected due to their secretive nature and the fact that persons who engage in these acts are rarely motivated to seek treatment for their behaviour.

A number of paraphilias are difficult to clarify. Some seem closely linked to fetishism but instead of body parts, body discharges take on erotic significance. Coprophilia, for example, involves erotic fascination with feces; klismaphilia with enemas; urophilia with urine; and mysophilia with filth. These stimuli may excite or be used for orgasm. Soiling others—by urinating or defecating on them-can also serve sadomasochistic purposes and is sometimes seen in assaults and rape situations.

Some paraphilias may have a sexual goal that is not immediately obvious. For example, pyromania (fire setting) and kleptomania (stealing for excitement) are thought to sometimes represent sexualized activities and thereby qualify as paraphilias.

Frotteurism (or toucherism) is a paraphilia that involves sexual gratification or arousal by rubbing against or fondling an unsuspecting, nonconsenting person. The frotteur acts on urges to touch, rub, or fondle usually in crowed places, often accompanied by fantasies of having sex with the singled-out person. Contact is brief to avoid detection.

Finally, the 20th century has brought a host of

telephone scatologia, or efforts to seek sexual gratification by making obscene telephone calls. Anonymity and escape from detection are enhanced in use of this media for contact.

Causal models and treatments: Several key observations and assumptions should be noted before addressing the etiology and treatment of sexual disorders. First, contemporary sexologists have had little success in identifying specific causal factors and in designing and implementing successful treatment modalities. Such a state is due, in part, to limited theoretical models and problematic methodology. Criticism of existing causal models have been in terms of their myopic and/ or reductionistic focus. In other words, most theories have focused solely on cognitive/emotional, behavioural, or environmental elements rather than on how all three elements interact and affect an individual's sexual identity. Another factor may be methodological problems, e.g., the difficulty in forming operational definitions for, and measuring such abstract concepts as, gender identity or sexual orientation. A more important and subtle point however, is the view that by separating the range of sexual behaviours into specific categories and calling these "abnormal," we are, by this process alone, not asking the critical questions about how sexual identity and orientation develop as a phenomena. Instead, we are caught up in treating our categorizations as if they are real and true medical diseases or abnormalities. In fact, it appears that sexual expression can vary greatly and lies on a continuum. Even though experience and socialization can affect the location of one's position on the continuum, we know very little about how individuals get to a particular place on the continuum in the first place. Biological theories have predominated as causes of sexual disorders. The specific biological determinant or process would have to be in the male and not female structures. No absolute causative biological mechanisms have been identified. Most behavioural scientists see very little value in the psychoanalytic or psychodynamic theories. Both deficient psychosexual development and Oedipal fixations have been used to account for sexual disorders. Repressed hostility is though to be at the roots of most paraphilias and the disorder allows a symbolic acting out of these repressed urges.

Learning theory models emphasize classical conditioning or associative learning linking sexual arousal with previously neutral objects or situations, masturbation becoming a key activity for this linking to occur. Learning theory seems to account for some paraphilias and for some portion of the sexual disorders but it lack sex sufficient empirical power and predictability.

As mentioned previously, treatments for the paraphilias and other sexual disorders are very ineffective and positive effects seem to be confined to highly motivated clients with milder forms of the disorders. Biological treatments essentially attempt to dull or reduce sexual drive. The behaviour therapies utilize counter-conditioning and desensitization methods. Various forms of group therapies (structured in a self-help manner) seem to be effective with the motivated client.

Sexual addiction: How far do normal sexual activity levels extend? Where do we draw the line for pathological levels of sexual activity? Again, changes in social values have defined different patterns and points on the sexual activity continuum as pathological at different times. As a matter of fact, lack of precision in defining this category and the subjective nature of judgments resulted in the elimination of sexual addiction from the paraphilias in the DSM-III-R edition.

The terms "sexual addiction" and "sexual compulsion" began to appear in the scientific and clinical literature in the 1970s. They soon became popular terms to describe individuals who seemed obsessed with sexual behaviour, i.e., nymphomaniacs, etc. Usually, sexual activity had to reach a level where it interfered with their job, relationships, career, or even their health. The behaviour was often described as uncontrolled sexual behaviour but functional analysis showed that it tended to lower anxiety states and probably helped enhance self-esteem and the sense of power and control.

Critics of the use of these concepts or diagnostic categories argued that they lacked precision and behavioural clarity, that they were often unreliable, and full of subjective judgements. Critics pointed out that the concepts did not fit our knowledge of the addictions nor of the compulsive processes. Furthermore, they were often applied to gay men with many partners and thus seemed discriminatory.

Supporters of this category argued that frequency was not the issue, rather one had to look at the purpose and meaning to the individual as critical components. Here, seeking out transient relationships in an indiscriminate manner certainly had the ring of self-defeating and self-destructive patterns of behaviour that qualified as paraphilias.

At this point, however, sexual addiction is an historical term.

Rape: Rape (Latin, "to seize") or the actual act of seizing a person by physical force or threat is an extreme form of sexual aggression and coercion. Rape is technically a legal term but it can be viewed from a psychological perspective. Current definitions of rape have extended the violation to deliberate intrusion into the emotional, physical, or rational integrity of the individual and even debasement through voyeurism ("visual rape"). Legally, rape is divided into statutory (seduction of a minor) and forcible seizure of an unwilling partner overage 18. Recent attention has been focused on "date rape" or the use of coercion by dates, acquaintances or even boyfriends. The victims are almost always women. No woman is entirely safe from rape. Almost 100,000 rape are reported each year but estimates are the majority of rapes go unreported. Most occur outside or in the victim's home. National studies have found that the incidence of rape has increased more rapidly than any other type of violent crime.

There are many factors and levels of causation to rape. Certainly, cultural and subcultural attitudes towards women and about men contribute to the setting for rape. Psychological studies of rapists have identified some broad typologies of rapists. These types were derived from psychological examination of rape cases. In none of these cases was it found that rape was motivated by sexual satisfaction. All the cases were characterized by a predominance of power motive or anger. This lead to the classification or rapists as (1) power assertive types (intimidation and control), (2) power reassurance types (to compensate for an under lying sense of weakness and inadequacy), (3) anger-retaliation type (rage, hatred, and violence predominate), and anger-excitation rape (the pathological sadist).

Prediction of rape from psychological profiles is not possible even though a proportion of rapists are obviously disturbed. The literature in this area is replete with instances of rape, in which, prior to the attack, the rapist had given no hint whatsoever of being a dangerous person. Conviction rates for rape are low and treatment or therapeutic interventions have generally been ineffective and disappointing. In addition to the need to develop adequate predictive and therapeutic measures for rapists, there is a tremendous need to improve treatments for the traumatized victims of these violent crimes.

Heterosocial skills are a major component of sexual behaviour is not a new idea. Basing their procedures on the idea that sexual deviation, particularly homosexuality, is a result of fear or avoidance of the opposite sex, therapists of many persuasions have encouraged and taught appropriate social behaviours in a heterosexual context. Many have reported this strategy to be successful. Other therapists and clinical researchers working with procedures to change patterns of sexual arousal have noted the insufficiency of such efforts alone in establishing functional heterosexual behaviour in many cases. Even if successful sexual behaviour is established, many patients are still unable to meet, date, or successfully relate to persons of the opposite sex. Many of the therapists working on this problem have concluded that deficits in social skills in heterosexual situations are responsible for these failures and that there is a necessity of assessing heterosocial skills. In a general review of the literature concerned with training in social skills, Hersen and Eisler point out that many forms of treatment have implicitly acknowledged the existence of poor interpersonal adjustment but have focused their treatment efforts for the most part on relatively unstructured attempts to improve socializing through therapeutic milieus or group therapy. The behavioural approach to treatment, as applied to training in social skill, has emphasized a more precise analysis of the verbal and nonverbal components of adequate social skills in treatment, but this emphasis requires a more precise assessment of behaviours comprising social skills than was heretofore available. Moreover, Eisler, Hersen, Miller, and Blanchard have noted that effective and necessary social skills may differ depending on the situation or circumstance. Thus skills necessary for heterosocial situations may differ from social skills necessary in work-related situations.

There are at least three facets of heterosocial skills: (1) a set of social behaviours is necessary to initiate relationships with the opposite sex; (2) a chain of social and interpersonal behaviours precedes sexual behaviour; (3) the maintenance of heterosocial relationships may require behaviours different from the first two facets.

The assessment of heterosocial behaviour has not progressed far. Current assessment procedures are directed at only the first step in the chain of heterosocial behaviour—initiating a relationship. Almost all these assessment procedures have been developed in contrived situations, usually involving some sort of role playing. The emphasis thus far has been on direct behavioural assessment in a contrived situation although self-report and, in one instance, physiological assessment of heterosocial skills have also occurred. Behavioural assessment in the natural environment has occurred infrequently although one interesting example will be cited later. Self-report or behaviour records similar to those used in assessing sexual arousal behaviour in the natural environment have also been used to assess social skills. Physiological assessment has noted occurred in the natural environment.

To date the bulk of the work on development of assessment procedures for heterosocial skills has come from analogue studies on college students with dating problems., rather than patients. However, in attempting to determine behaviours that differentiate people with adequate social skills from those with inadequate skills, most studies have been unable to identify specific behaviours. These studies have found that overall ratings of heterosocial skills discriminate high-frequency daters from low-frequency daters, but the identification of specific behaviours has proved elusive. In these and other studies the only valid assessment of heterosocial skills seemed to be trained raters' judgment of overall social skills while observing interactions in contrived situations.

In these contrived situations self-reports of social skills and other aspects of heterosocial functioning such as "confidence" were often collected in addition to direct behavioural observation carried this one step farther and had male subjects record frequency and duration of contacts with women outside the contrived situation in the natural environment. They also demonstrated that physiological assessments of anxiety in social situations, in this case simple pulse rate, showed improvement after training in social skills,indicating that assessment of this response modality may be useful. Most of this research investigated the social behaviour of male subjects only, have recently begun investigating hetero-social behaviour in females.

In a clinical setting Barlow, Abel, Blanchard, Bristow, and Your have constructed a behavioural checklist that differntiates competent heterosocial males from socially incompetent male patients with sexual problems. To develop this scale, high school ad college males judged socially attractive by a panel of popular females in their schools were videotaped interacting with female research assistants. Ten patients with sexually deviant behaviours who reported and were judged to be heterosocially inadequate were also videotaped interacting with a female. Behaviours in three categories—form of conversation, affect, and voice—significantly discriminated the adequate from the inadequate males. *Voice* quality was rated on loudness, pitch, and inflection whereas *affect* was rated on the basis of facial expression, eye contact, and laughter. Judgment of the appropriate *form* of conversation was based on whether the male initiated conversation, responded to the females' vocalization, prevented uncomfortably long silences in the conversation, and showed interest in his partner. Responses as defined in the behaviour checklist could be reliably scored by trained raters. For purposes of the original validation, patients entered a room and were instructed to engage the female confederate in conversation with the ultimate purpose of asking for a date. The interaction lasted approximately four to five minutes and was divided into 30-second blocks. If any inappropriate behaviour occurred within a 30-second block, the block was rated inappropriate. For further information on the use of this behavioural checklist, see Barlow et al.

Like other investigations using nonpatient populations, this scale was constructed around a contrived situation and is appropriate for males only. Direct behavioural assessment in the natural environment, using this checklist should present no technical problems, since the transference of the raters into the natural environment would be the only change required. Such an assessment in the natural environment would be necessary only if the initiation of heterosocial relationships occurred in a public setting. By posing as a bar patron, Maletzky surreptitiously observed homosexuals initiating relationships in a gay bar. In this case the observations were used as an assessment of the effectiveness of treatment. This type of assessment presents obvious ethical problems, however, which is most likely why it has been utilized infrequently. A proper assessment can only be done surreptitiously, since the presence of known raters would make the measures extremely obtrusive. Current-day ethical standards in either research or clinical settings preclude this type of observation without the informed consent of the patient. Hersen and Eisler have suggested that it might be possible to circumvent this ethical barrier by obtaining the subjects' permission to make these types of observation without telling them the specific time. Investigations along these lines are sorely needed, if only to determine the validity of assessment in contrived situations.

Similarly, assessment procedures to investigate social behaviour related to initiation of genital contact are lacking despite the frequent clinical observation of deficits in this area. Even married couples often report "shyness," that is, deficits in the types of behaviours necessary to initiate sexual relationships.

Deviation in gender role: The final component of sexual behaviour is confused gender identity or deviation in gender role, which refers to some degree of incongruence between one's biological and genetic sex and the behaviour accompanying that sex as defined by a given culture.

Society is more familiar with the concepts of masculinity and femininity than with the other aspects of sexual behaviour mentioned in this chapter, and yet these concepts are among the most difficult to measure or assess. The familiarity and pervasiveness of maleness and femalenes ensured an early interest in these concepts from the psychological point of view. Still, the ease with which people identify and discuss male and female behaviour may be responsible for the lack of development of precise definitions. The growth of interest in gender identity and gender role behaviour is owing to two recent developments. The phenomenon of transsexualism, in which a biologically and genetically normal person thinks, feels, and behaves as if he or she were a member of the opposite sex and often requests sex reassignment surgery, has rearoused interest in the development of gender identity. Second,the emergence of women's role in our society as a political issue has aroused interest in sex role stereotypes that can be broken down into gender-specific behaviours and attitudes, or the more common terms, "masculinity" and "femininity". The discovery that transsexualism is a clinical entity and not merely a defense mechanism highlighted gender role behaviour and raised some intriguing questions onther relation of gender role behaviour to sexual problems, particularly sexual deviations. Why are gender role deviations associated with some sexual arousal patterns, such as homosexuality and transvestism, and not with others? Why are some homosexuals effeminate and others not? Is femininity in females the same as femininity in males. Is femininity in males related to pedophilia? Does society tolerate masculine women more than feminine men? These and other questions require precise assessments of the degree of gender role deviations.

The discovery that gender role deviation is related to outcome in the treatment of some sexual deviations has aroused even more interest. Bieber, Bieber, Dain, Dince, Drellich, Grand, Grundlach, Kremer, Wilbur, and Bieber, in reporting that up to 50 percent of certain subgroups of homosexuals achieved some heterosexual orientation after psychoanalysis, observed that no subjects responded positively to psychoanalysis if there was evidence of gender role deviation in their background. Marks, Gelder, and Bancroft reported encouraging success in treating a group of transvestites who had no gender role deviations, but among those transvestites who had some degree of gender role deviation, there was no recovery. These studies, from quite different approaches, suggest the importance of gender role deviations as a factor in sexual deviations.

Early attempts to measure gender identity are of some historical interest. They consisted mostly of questionnaires requiring the subject to state interests or preferred activities. One of the best known tests was the M-F test of Terman and Miles, which consisted of a number of different questions and exercises, including inkblot associations. Variations on this test have included the well-known scale on the MMPI and the femininity scale of the California Psychological Inventory. Scales of this type have proved useless in assessing gender identity or gender role deviations. Major problems with these scales were their vagueness and the cultural temporal relativity of the questions. For instance, on the California Personality Inventory scale a question, "I would like to be soldier" must be answered in the affirmative to score as masculine.

Some investigators have suggested that the assessment of gender role deviations such as femininity in males requires a different instrument from the usual M-F test since some items would be unique to feminine males. Thus extremely effeminate males or tansexuals, rather than women, should be the referent group. Although the scale constructed by Freund *et al.* is very useful, the similarities and differences (other than the obvious ones) between effeminate males and females or masculine females and males have yet to be identified. The development of reliabie and valid measuring instruments is required. To date, instruments to assess gender role have been developed in both the self-report and behavioural response systems. The physiological response system does not seem relevant to this component of sexual behaviour. However, there is recent evidence of the possible biochemical nature of gender role deviation. This evidence is important and requires assessment. Unlike other components, behavioural measures of gender role can occur in the natural environment as well as in contrived situations.

A body-image scale for evaluating transsexuals has been reported by Lindgren and Pauly. This scale measures a person's satisfaction with he physical appearance of his different body parts. Transsexuals are typically very dissatisfied with their actual physical appearance, particularly in the genital area, and thus an assessment of this factor is useful whether one is treating transsexuals by surgical means or by modifying gender role behaviours. However, the scale has not as yet been widely used. In our laboratory the card sort measure, described in the section above on self-report of sexual arousal, is also used to assess transsexual attitudes.

A second recent approach to measure deviation in gender role grows out of the developing interest in sex-role stereotypes and attempts to measure a person's affinity for one sex role or the either in nonpatient populations. Perhaps the best example of this type of questionnaire is a sex role inventory developed by Bem. Her inventory threats masculinity and femininity as two independent dimensions so that it is possible to characterize a person as either masculine, feminine, or androgynous, which represents the positive aspects of both sex roles. Typical masculine personality items the subject may choose in this sex role inventory are "aggressive" and "ambitious". Typical feminine items are "affectionate" and "cheerful". This scale is satisfactory on most psychometirc dimensions, but it was not designed to assess the degree of gender role deviations. However, it has been applied in our laboratories to transsexuals and other patients with gender role deviations and provides interesting information on sex role preference.

Behavioural measures: Assessment of gender-specific behaviour presents fewer technical problems than other sexual behaviour. Gender-specific behaviours tend to occur in any setting where behaviour is occurring at all, including sitting, standing, or walking. Two distinct methods for developing behavioural checklists for masculine and feminine behaviour are emerging, one for children and the other for adults. For children, the typical checklist for gender role behaviour is used in a contrived situation, usually a room set up with specific types of toys or other play activities previously determined to be feminine or masculine. This type of assessment has been in use for some time, beginning with Terman and Miles, and has occasionally been updated and revalidated by other investigators have conducted the most sophisticated analysis of toy preference and have reported high discriminant validity when testing masculine and feminine boys. Green and others are using this measure in a variety of studies to assess the effects of treating gender role deviations in effeminate boys.

The ready availability of observers, usually parents or teachers, should ensure an easy extension of assessment of gender role behaviour into the natural environment. Such assessment will be facilitated by the development of a variety of behaviour checklists that go beyond play activities in children. For instance, Hanaway isolated a specific behaviour the way in which one carries books and discovered that it accurately discriminated high school and college students. He then followed this behaviour down through progressively younger age groups and found that the behaviour discriminated males and females very well through the fourth grade but broke down in the third grade and below. These data indicate that assessments of 9- and 10-year-old children for gender-specific behaviour could include the book-carrying task.

Attempts to develop behaviour checklists or rating scales of gender-specific behaviour in adults are limited, despite the fact that "clinical impressions" are in abundance. Some work in identifying gender-specific behaviours in adults has begun recently. This work has emerged from two sources although the goals of pinpointing sex differences of gender-specific behaviours are similar. The first area of work originated in the investigations of Birdwhistell and Argyle. A good example of this line of research is a study reported by Weitz. As a social psychologist, Weitz approaches the problem of sex role stereotypes and normal sex role development in the manner of Bem. For example, Weitz noted, while studying noverbal behaviour associated with interactions, that women elicit more nonverbal warmth than men and that women in general are more responsive and attentive to the other interactant. Weitz's working assumption is that the microprocesses of interaction reveal the macrostructure of sex roles. Although this type of investigation is not intended to have any direct relevance on the assessment or treatment of sexual problems, alterations of deviations in gender role must eventually consider the full range gender-specific behaviour, including social behaviour, to assess adequately deviation in gender role.

Approaching the assessment of gender-specific from the view-point of sexual problems, Schatzberg, Westfall, Blumetti, and Birk devised a quantitative rating of effeminacy for use with males. Noting that deviations in gender role were an important component of many sexual deviations, they constructed a comprehensive list of 67 items scored on a simple yes/no basis. The items were assumed to break down effeminate behaviour in males into discrete behavioural fragments so that the presence or absence of the behaviour could be easily scored. The checklist was then tested on a nonpatient population of heterosexual and homosexual males. Items in the area of speech, gait (Does he move sinuously?), mouth movements (Does he purse his lips when he speaks?), and the like were examples of items on the checklist. Seventeen of the 67 items were not scored for any of the 32 subjects in the initial study. Subjects were interviewed during a 15-minute, semistructured interview. After the interview two rates completed the scale. Although the correlation of the total scores of the raters was high, the interrater agreement was low at chance level. This interrater agreement is not surprising because raters could not score behaviours until after the interview was over. The homosexual group scored somewhat more effeminate with a mean of 7.0 on this scale. which compared to approximately 3.5 for the hetero-sexual group of males. The fact that one is more likely to find gender role deviations in homosexuals than in heterosexuals suggests that the scale has some discriminate validity, although given the low interrater agreement, the nature of the discriminating factors are not clear. It is probable that an overall impression of femininity was being rated. In addition, the scale seems to have a very small range of effectiveness. Our of 67 items, the authors scored a total of five through nine as being mildly effeminate. Nevertheless, the scale is a breakthrough of sorts in that it is the first of its kind and deserves further investigation. An advantage of this scale is that it need not be administered in the contrived situation of a semistructured interview but can theoretically be administered in any setting, including surreptitious settings in the natural environment. The investigators tested the scale in a variety of social contexts that occurred in four encounter groups. They found a wide variability in ratings of effeminacy, which they correlated with emotional responses such as anxiety of anger.

For the past several years a checklist of masculine-feminine motoric behaviour has been in use in our laboratories, particularly for the assessment of deviations in gender role. This checklist pinpoint gender-specific aspects of sitting, standing, and walking. For instance, males tend to sit with the lower back and buttocks away from the back of a hard-backed chair and cross their legs with he ankle resting on the opposite knee. Females, on the other hand, sit with their lower back an buttocks close to the back of the chair and cross their legs with one knee resting on the other. Interrater agreement is 92.5 percent for walking, 100 percent of sitting, 97.45 percent for standing.

Sexuality: As late as the early 1900s, it was common to "explain" human sexual behaviour in terms of instincts. For example Freud postulated a sexual instinct and "explained" people's sex drive in terms of an instinctual energy he called libido. Gradually instinct theories have been recognized as weak hypothetical constructs and replaced by more detailed models of the biological, psychological, and social causes of motivation and behaviour. Current theories of sexuality recognize that sexual behaviour involves multiple components that interact complexly. The most basic elements of this multifactor model of sexual behaviour are the reflex mechanism that cause vaginal lubrication, penile erection, other genital responses, and orgasm. These reflexes influence and are influenced by both instrumental learning and classical conditioning, which in turn are affected by the type of home, community, and culture in which a person lives. Finally, as children develop more cognitive capacities, they can increasingly plan unique and creative ways of directing their sexual experiences.

Reflexes: The sexual responses of the genitals are mediated by several reflex centers located in the lower spinal cord. The most basic way to activate the sexual reflexes is by touch to the genitals. Nerves connecting the genitals to the spinal reflex centers respond to touch as the unconditioned stimulus that activates them—without the need for any prior conditioning. The reflex mechanisms then activate all the genital changes associated with sexual arousal, such as vaginal lubrication, penile erection, and—after enough stimulation—orgasm. They also send signals to and respond to signals from the brain. The connections with the brain allow sexual responses to influence and be influenced by learning, memory, and thought.

The sex reflexes operate from birth, but the hormonal changes of puberty lead to increasing sexual sensitivity and spontaneous responses in the genitals. The reflexive and inborn facets of sexual behaviour are not, by themselves, adequate for assuring intercourse or successful reproduction.

Considerable learning is needed for an individual to become sexually active. Since learning is influenced significantly by individual, social, and cultural variables—and each person has a unique history of learning experiences—there is considerable variability in human sexual activities both within and between societies.

Perception and instrumental learning: The neural pathways that connect the reflex centers in the lower spine to the brain connect with the sensory centers in the cerebral cortex, allowing people to perceive many types of sensations from the genitals. Some of these perceptions enter into long-term memory and influence later thoughts and actions.

In addition, some of the neural inputs from the genitals innervate the pleasure and pain centers in the brain, such that certain types of genital stimulation are experienced as pleasant, while other types are painful. Through instrumental learning (also known as operant conditioning), people usually learn to repeat those activities that are followed by pleasurable, rewarding experiences and avoid those followed by aversive sensations. We learn to do things that instrumental in attaining pleasure (such as those things leading to orgasm) and avoiding pain (or reinforcement) and punishment help assure that most people learn sexual practices that are instrumental in attaining sexual pleasure—which, before the advent of birth control, often served the biological function or promoting pregnancy and the reproduction of the species.

The more rewarding—and less aversive—a person's experiences with sex, the more positive associations and memories the person tends to have about sex; and this usually translates to greater sexual motivation—or "sex drive"—if there are no biological problems that detrimentally affect the sexual response systems.

Classical conditioning: The sexual reflex is among the reflexes that are capable of being conditioned via classical conditioning (also known as Pavlovian conditioning). Namely, when a neutral stimulus is paired repeatedly with the unconditioned stimulus of appropriate touch to the genitals, that neutral stimulus gradually becomes a conditioned stimulus capable of eliciting the sexual reflex. In common parlance, these conditioning stimuli are called "erotic stimuli" or "sexual turn-ons". Usually, the more frequently that an erotic stimulus or turn-on has been paired with the unconditioned stimulus to touch to the genitals, the more capable that conditioned stimulus is of eliciting sexual responses-unless a person has so many negative associations with or biological problems affecting sex that they suppress the sexual response.

Through classical conditioning, almost any stimulus that is frequently paired with and is predictive of the sexual arousal can become an erotic stimulus or sexual turn-on. The specific stimuli that people respond to as sexually exciting differ from person to person, depending on each individual's prior sexual experiences. Many people learn to respond to pictures or fantasies of nude bodies as erotic stimuli, if these have been paired with masturbation or sexual interactions in the past. Some come to find "talking dirty" to be sexually arousing, if such talk has been a common part of their exciting sexual experiences. Although many people would be offended by vulgar language and do not understand how anyone could find it sexually exciting, the principles of classical conditioning allow us to understand that almost any stimulus can become an erotic stimulus or sexual turn-on, for those individuals who have experience it in conjunction with sexual excitement.

When people learn to imagine their erotic stimuli (in the absence of any external stimuli), they gain the ability to fantasize about their turn-ons. Since having sexual fantasies is often pleasurable, many people learn this cognitive activity—unless guilt or other bad feelings punish such fantasies. Some people cultivate elaborate sexual fantasies because of the pleasure and sexual arousal that they bring.

Nerves that connect the cortex to the sexual reflex mechanisms in the lower spinal cord allow cortical activity—such as seeing or fantasizing about sexual turn-ons—to activate the sexual reflexes. This is called psychogenic stimulation of the sexual reflexes, since the excitation is psychological in origin. For some people, psychogenic stimulation only produces a mild sexual response, such as slight vaginal lubrication or partial penile erection; but in other people, the response can be quite strong, sometimes leading to orgasm. There is a great deal of variation among people in the strength of these psychogenic responses, these differences being due to the number and intensity of positive and negative learning experiences that any given individual has had with sexuality.

During sexual intercourse, fantasies and psychogenic sexual stimulation can add to the total excitement that enhances the sexual response. Fantasies also serve to distract people from some of the stimuli that can inhibit the sexual response-e.g., guild about sexual activities, fears of not being attractive enough to one's partner, or fears about the adequacy of one's sexual performance.

The sexual reflexes can be inhibited by aversive conditioning. Any of a variety of sex-related stimuli can become associated with fear, worry, or anxiety—depending on each individual's unique history of classical conditioning. For one persons, fears of becoming pregnant can interfere with the sexual of pregnancy. Fear of not pleasing one's partner, not beingable to have orgasms, or anything else can inhibit the sex reflex. Given the pervasive social attention to physical attractiveness—especially for females—some peoples feel anxious that their partner will not think their body is attractive enough.

Nonsocial and scial learning: Some learning is clearly social, as when we watch other people's actions—perhaps via movies or videos—and learn from them. However, sexual learning may occur alone, as when a child explores touching his or her body, discovers masturbation, and pairs certain fantasies with sexual activities. But even these relatively nonsocial activities, done in private, are usually not devoid of social influence. For example, the child's frequency of masturbation is influenced by the degree to which the parents accept or punish masturbation. Each individual's choice of fantasy images used during masturbation is often affected by prior social experiences.

Social learning theory emphasizes that we learn a great deal from observing the actions and listening to the words of others, who are called models. Although sexual intercourse is usually not done publicly in our society, people learn about sex in private from observing and listening to their sexual partners. People also learn the sexual activities of symbolic models presented in magazines, books, movies, TV, and videos. In addition, there are many sex-related activities—such as meeting, becoming intimate, and suggesting sexual activities—that are modeled more often in public than is sexual behaviour per se. Once information is acquired by observing others, people may later attempt similar actions. The degree to which they fully adopt the behaviour depends on how instrumental it is in bringing them rewarding effects. Did a sexual position modeled in a video bring pleasure or complaints from one's partner?

Not only do people learn the physical activities of sex by observing and listening to others, they learn how others talk about sex and play out sexual roles. Patterns of talk and action are often called "scripts", and sexual scripts are involved at every stage from meeting a potential partner to making love. For example, there are countless opening lines a person can use to meet another, and research indicates that women are more discerning among them that are men. Men like almost all types of opening lines that women use to strike up a conversation; but women tend to like direct and innocuous lines and be turned off by cute-flippant lines from men. There are the countless scripts for dealing with sex, and they vary from society to society—from subculture to subculture. This can creat confusion when people move from one social sphere to another or try to become intimate with someone from a different subculture.

Cognitive and social psychology: Cognitive psychology adds another level of complexity to the multifactor model of sexuality. Our perceptual experience enters inputs from all sense modalities into thought and memory. Our thoughts are composed mostly of visual imagery, sounds, and the inner words we "hear" in our minds as we think to ourselves. Whereas sexy pictures can influence our visual sexual fantasies, the sexual scripts we learn tend to influence the inner words we use to think about sex. When teens see TV shows or movies in which certain lines or scripts lead to sexually exciting outcomes, they may find themselves rehearing those words in their minds and then using parts of combinations of those scripts with others.

Social psychology stresses how much each individual is influenced by his or her position in society. Two people living in the same country—but exposed to different subsets of the multiple cultures possible within a society have access to different models, media, books, videos—which provide them with different ideas about sexual conduct. Some obtain vast amounts of information about sex, birth control, and relationships, while others obtain little. From each person's unique perspective on life, each develops personal views and opinions. As a result, two people can interpret the same event very differently: Two people can see the same erotic movie, and one calls it interesting while the other calls it repulsive pornography.

Cognitive and social psychology emphasize the importance of people's cognitive processes in interpreting their situations, creating unique and personal plans of action and making novel contributions to their social interactions. People are not passive receptacles, only being shaped by society. They are active, creative makers of their own social lives. They modify and creatively reconstruct the scripts and action patterns learned from society, producing their own unique contributions and social constructions. Creativity stems from many sources, two of which, of example, are fantasy and problem solving. People often invent creative fantasies, involving images and scripts, that can lead to plans for doing sexual activities they have never done before. People may consciously attempt to create a special sexual experience that is uniquely their own. Through that creative recombination of different scripts, fantasies, and novel ideas, people can construct sexual plans and actions that differ from anything they have ever seen used by others. Though perhaps no radically different from their culture, their actions are creative variations. Problems often cause people to search for creative solutions. When people face a problem, such as increasing boredom with sex after 10 years of marriage, the problem may stimulate creative efforts to devise novel and interesting sexual experiences.

As millions of creative people invent novel ideas and share them with others, the total contributions have their impact in changing the sexual practices of the larger society. Many new ideas are lost after being tried a few times, but others (usually the most rewarding ones) spread and become widely popular. Magazines and books may help popularize a sexual position or fantasy. People also change their society by voting, for example using the ballot to express their values about abortion, nude beaches, pornography, and other sex-related topics. By showing how people's values and creative thoughts affect their society, cognitive and social psychology empower people to take a stronger role in changing social conditions related to sexuality, gender and reproductive rights.

Sex drive: Psychology used to conceive of behaviour is a function of drives and people today still talks about sex drive and libido. But with the development of multifactor models of behaviour, the concept of drive is now seen as simplistic. People's desires and motivations for sex result from the multiple causes, some biological and others social-psychological in origin.

Testosterone heightens sexual motivation in males—and probably in females. (Normally women have small amounts of testosterone in their bodies that are adequate for promoting sexual interest.) Good health tends to facilitate sexual desire and pleasure; whereas illness, depression, drug abuse, and other biomedical factors tend to reduce sexual motivation. Also, the more prior rewards and less prior punishment a person has experienced with sex, the stronger the person's sexual interest and motivation tends to be. Punishment related to sex leads to inhibition that can reduce a person's sexual motivation. The more sexual turn-ons and fantasies a persons developed (via classical conditioning), the more likely his or her sexual interest will be piqued by numerous events of everyday life that might not be perceived as sexual by another [who has not eroticized those stimuli]. Also, the more sexual scripts a person has learned, the more the person tends to think and act in sexual ways.

There is no single "normal" level of sexual desire. Two people with high sexual desire may be very happy with their sexual life having sexual interactions every day; and two people with low sexual desire may have an equally satisfactory sex life, *engaging in intercourse twice a month.* Sexual desire is most likely to be a problem in a couple's relationship when the two have discrepant sexual desire—one wanting sex much more than the other.

Sexual orientation: Although many people think that there are only two types of sexual orientation—heterosexual and homosexual—the issue is much more complex. There is a continuum of positions between these two extremes with bisexuality lying in the middle. The definitions of these three terms set the stage for understanding the whole continuum. "Heterosexuals" are people whose primary erotics, psychological, emotional, and social interest is in members of the other sex—even though that interest may not be overtly expressed, "Homosexuals" are people whose primary erotic, psychological, emotional, and social interest is in members of the same sex—even though that interest may not be overtly expressed, "Bisexuals" have both of these capacities.

Alfred Kinsey was the first sex researcher to provide a method of describing sexual orientation on a continuum, with 0 being pure heterosexual, 3 being bisexual, and 6 being pure homosexual. People who are at position one are mostly heterosexual, but have some homosexual orientation. Each higher number represents greater homosexual orientation. Kinsey and his coresearchers actually devised two separate scales. one measured overt sexual experience, and the other psychosexual reactions, such as erotic feelings, emotions, and fantasies. In most cases a person's position on one scale is the same as on the other scale. However, there are cases in which people's overt sexual behaviour does not completely parallel his or her psychosexual reactions. For example, some homosexuals can respond sexually to the other sex, even though they find that their emotional and psychological attachment is to the same sex. Also, a person can be homosexual and never engage in sexual relations with a member of the same sex.

Sex roles: Several definitions and further distinctions need to be made to avoid confusion. The first distinction can be made between sex and gender. In 1979, Unger attempted to clarify the distinction between sex and gender for the discipline of Psychology. She argued that sex should be limited to the biological bases of producing the two primary genders: the presence of XX or XY chromosomes, hormonal output from the gonads, internal and external reproductive anatomy, and secondary sex characteristics. Gender on the other hand is what culture does with the evidence of biological sex. Ultimately the culture creates expected behaviour patterns or styles which are deemed gender specific. A second distinction can be made between sex roles and sex role stereotypes. The former include the actual behaviours of males and females which have considerable variability. The latters are oversimplified socially shared perceptions of idealized male" or "female" actions, perceptions which usually allow little variability. Third, sexuality differs from sex roles. The roles are overt behaviours of many kinds, including sexuality, linked to "maleness" and "femalenes." Sexuality is the behaviour directly associated with having sex or being sexually involved. Fourth, gender identity, one's sense of oneself as essentially "male" or "female" may or may not be reflected in one's roles or one's sexuality. Fifth, gender schemes are the cognitive constructs used to conceptualize "male" or "femal" roles or identity, and, although held very deeply by the person, may not be congruent with his or her behaviour.

Gender differences, defined as distinctions that can be made between maleness and femaleness or between males and females themselves, are a problematic category. Psychologists often find it hard to decide how much difference is a true difference. We often confuse differences in perceptions or constructs of sex roles with differences in actual behaviour of males and females. Yet decisions about "differences" often lead to broad public policy decisions.

Defining and measuring sex roles in polarized terms (i.e., "male" vs "female") may be erroneous. According to Rabin, the idea that there are only two biological sexes needs reexamination. There are numerous examples from biology that indicate more possibilities than just two complementary sexes. We find hermaphronditic species which contain both reproductive capacities within one body, and even one all-female species of whiptail lizard which reproduces partheogenetically. There are large numbers of coral reef fishes and tropical sand fishes which change sex. The popular polarization of the enormous range of human variability into two boxes at opposing ends of the human spectrum may be the consequence of normative thinking in the social sciences added to our penchant for creating dualities by ignoring the overlapping frequency distribution curves for male and female performance. Even when a statistically significant sex difference in performance in math skill or verbal skills can be demonstrated, this larger overlap between distributions means that the individuals whose performance falls within the overlap area cannot be distinguished on the basis of gender. Many females excel in math. Many males do poorly in math but excel in verbal skills. Differences that emerge are far more likely to be individual differences than actual gender differences separating all women from all men. So the most useful approach may be to think of and to measure maleness and femaleness on a continuum.

Confusion among these terms and models leads to negative results for science and for individuals. Conceptualizations of sex roles have been a function of philosophy, history, economics, and politics. Awareness that sex roles exist, and are influential, and that this occurs at all times in life, has also been a function of those four forces. These influences quietly shape the choice of problems to investigate and research projects to pursue. Most scientists in a given field accept some view of the world that dominates their field and choose problems accordingly. Driven by a need for cognitive consistency, individuals adopt the new view as "natural". In a world at war, for example, the role of a man is seen as that of a warrior, "naturally", and the role of a woman "naturally" becomes that of a worker/mother; after a return to peace, the woman may be "naturally" redefined as mother (only) while the now suddenly "nonwarlike" male is redefined as worker. Theories of adjustment, development, and mental health are quick to conform to the demands of the belief system and historical situation. Social psychology has made it clear that even radical shifts in ideas and behaviour are accepted to maintain thinking consistency, provided motivation is high enough. Researchers in human development are not immune to these general laws. We study what seems important at the time.

Gender role development across the life span: Early views of sex role development considered masculine and feminine roles are biologically based and, once established in childhood, consistent throughout the life span. The testing movement provided the impetus to quantify and validate such views. Masculinity and femininity were conceptualized as marking the two extreme endpoints of a continuum. Individuals were assumed to be optimally adjusted if their biological sex and their sex role identity were the same. An individual who deviated from a prescribed sex role was seen as one whose psychosexual development was inadequate, rather than as possibly a person who was flexible in meeting changing environmental demands. This view reflected the Freudian approach which depicted sex role identification in terms of resolution of the Oedipal conflict. Such a resolution involved the identification of a boy with his father and the girl, in a somewhat more circuitous way, with her mother. The possible learned nature of sex roles came to the forefront with the advent of social learning theory, cognitive developmental theory, biologically oriented inquirics, anthropological investigation, and the life span approach.

Social learning theory: Whereas Freud and other functionalists implied that sex roles merely unfold out of an innate potential, the social learning theorists such as Bandura posited that such roles were learned via imitation and observation of parents and other adult models. Reinforcement then led to the establishment of behavioural patterns. Although changes in reinforcement contingencies allowed the possibility for sex role change, it was assumed that the sex types roles did not change significantly during one's life span. Modeling the behaviours of the same sex was thought to begin at a very early age and to be reinforced into adulthood. However, research that has focused on modeling of adult behaviour or global personality traits shared by parent and child has not found that children closely follow the behaviour or personality of the same-sex adult.

Cognitive developmental theory: A cognitive developmental approach such as Kohlberg's, held that the child's perception of sex role identification precedes sex appropriate behaviour. The child discovered that two sexes existed, thought about himself or herself as being a boy or a girl, considered differences between the sexes, and came to some fairly stable notions as to what "boy/man" versus "girl/woman" connoted. Some of the same behavioural factors that the social learning theorists proposed were also expected, except that cognitive identification with a same-sex parent preceded the modeling of behaviours in terms of observation and imitation. The cognitive developmentalists also assumed that both children and adults maintained a relatively consistent concept of themselves as male or female, and that the search for congruence between belies and behaviour led to the maintenance of appropriate roles. This view may be contrasted with the social learning view in which reward is the key to the persistence of sex appropriate behaviour. Both theoretical viewpoints, however, emphasize the establishment of such an identity early in life with consistency in adulthood.

The learning perspective on sex roles has also received a valuable contribution from the biological perspective of Money and Ehrhardt. These researchers have studied children who genetically, and on the basis of prenatal hormones, would have been expected to develop the gender identity of one sex but because of mishap (for example, structural damage or deformity of the genitals) were assigned to the opposite sex. Interview data collected from the families of such children indicated that seeming acceptance of the assigned sex and gender role identity development proceeded commensurate with the child's acceptance of assigned gender identity. While these studies are by no means conclusive, they do point out the overwhelming impact of socialization.

Anthropological investigations: Anthropological study has supported the learned nature of sex roles and has led to questioning the notion of consistent, appropriate behaviours for each gender. The large impact of culture on any given society's notion of what is appropriate male and female behaviour has been exemplified by Mead's comparison of three primitive societies. Both the men and women of the Arapesh tribe were described as being passive, nurturant, cooperative, and sensitive, traits perceived as feminine in American culture. The Mundugamore men and women were characterized as aggressive, suspicious, and uncaring, traits perceived as masculine in American culture. The Tchambuli men behaved in ways our society, typically defines as feminine while the women exhibited what we might define as stereotypical masculine traits. The importance of culture-specific specialization has been expounded in numerous articles and books with respect to more modern societies as well.

The anthropological perspective has been used by researchers such as Gutmann to explore the function of sex roles in terms of survival of the species. Cultural universals are presumed to reflect basic human propensities; their consistency is assumed to be of some importance in terms of survival. Proponents of the learning approach, which emphasizes socialization, view exceptions to cultural universals as evidence for the greater impact of environment on heredity. Opponents point out that a few exceptions do not make a case against biological mechanisms but rather show evolutionary change within some special environmental conditions.

Adult developmental theories: The life span approach to sex role development has been a relatively recent phenomenon. Neugarten, Gutmann, and Block explored changes in male and female role expectations during adulthood that were based upon social expectation and major developmental tasks. Block and Riegel viewed the manifestation of cultural sex roles as a function not only of biological demands and past learning experiences but of the nature of economic systems, the historical moment, and the philosophical system within which they are defined. Thus, sex roles in this perspective imply dynamic change based upon the individual change and the social and cultural climate.

Loevinger's milestones of ego development and their extrapolations to sex role development form the basis of Block's approach. In the earliest period, the main development concerns of the child are genderless, and identity constitutes a mere naming of gender: "I am a boy/girl." Later, conformity to learned patterns becomes the main task; this is reflected in the development of sex role stereotypes and sex role bifurcation. This conformist stage is followed by one of self-criticism based on comparison with an abstract ideal, thereby moderating the stereotypical role. With the advent of autonomy, individualization results are conflicts, aroused during the conformity and conscientious stages, are resolved. At this point, differentiation of sex role is said to occur. The highest, most integrated level of functioning finds the individual evolving a complex identity which combines aspiration, experience, and previously polarized traits. In sex role terms, this period is one of androgyny.

Hefner, Rebecca, and Oleshansky have proposed a life span approach to the development of sex role identity. Their hierarchical stages include: (1) global, undifferentiated sex roles; (2) polarized, or traditional musculine/feminine roles, and (3) transcendent roles which combine both masculinity and femininity. While the young child most likely has not defined a sex role and the adolescent most likely has overdefined it, the adult synthesizes roles into more complex wholes. For individuals who have "transcended" masculinity and feminity, psychological adjustment is no longer tied to these dichotomous sets of traits, or even the blend of androgyny. Unfortunately, the measurement of "transcendence" as distinct from androgyny has not yet been fully operationalized.

Garnets and Pleck have presented a concept called sex role strain analysis. Their viewpoint combines social learning and life span development. They feel that the ultimate harm of traditional sex roles is the devaluation an individual may experience if he or she does not conform to traditional standards set by sex role norms. Thus, strain results from discrepancy between the individual's self-perception and his or her perceptions of social expectations. Garnets and Pleck also measure the degree of salience of sex role characteristics for the individual.

Sinnott described a postformal theory of adult sex role development. A number of investigators have recently addressed the topic of "postformal" operationals, i.e., those structures of thought which are a stage more complex in organisation than Piaget's formal operations. More work on postformal, mature adult thought is being done, possibly since the idea of cognitive development beyond adolescence is an appealing one. The question of interest here is: How might formal and postformal operations be related to a life span model of sex role development? To address this question it is necessary to examine some aspects of postformal operations and the argument itself more closely. The argument is a postmodern one.

What kind of case is being made for a relation between cognitive development, especially formal and postformal operations, and sex roles? To oversimplify, it is the same type of case that Kohlberg makes about cognitive development and early sex role development and about cognitive and moral development. Social relations, of which sex roles and more development are examples, may be seen as based upon cognitive skills. As cognitive skills develop, the social relations can be understood and can become more complex, too. At those times, when the world can be known in a manner more complex than an abstract, formal one, roles also might be known in a way that is more complex. Having thought of the role in a complex way, one could then live it in a complex way.

How would roles be known in postformal terms? To answer this question, one must look at theories of postformal operations. According to Kramer, authors of these theories all state that postformal thought is: (1) a distinct stage, (2) which subsumes formal operations, and (3) which incorporates a relativistic view of truth. Generally, then, a postformal cognitive stage could underlie a view of sex roles in which roles are not absolute but are created relative to the actor. Some given formal structure of roles would be consciously chosen based on some belief system that is a subjective view of "trouth" from among a number of formal role structures. Further, what constitutes a given role would be known to be somewhat arbitrary and based partly on the perceiver's own experiences and resultant ideas of the role. The postformal concept of sex roles, then, includes a necessary subjectivity. It operates by laws like those of the new physics as described by Sinnott.

The role taken, or the role which one perceives that another takes, becomes what is agreed on by the persons in the interaction. The reality of the role is therefore determined by a system of beliefs held by the persons in the interaction. The individual is not in a roleless, underfined state, nor in possession of an absolute unchanging role, which is a permanent descriptor of one's identity. Rather he or she is constantly, perhaps even consciously, creating a flexible role definition in relation to individuals and circumstances in context. In the framework of Kelly's theory of personality, persons are always constructing a new social meaning for the self in the context of evolving social structures within a given society's institutions.

Role behaviours also may be seen as attempts to solve everyday life problems. Individuals learn to act in a way which helps them meet their goals. In the context of problem solving, which is a cognitive function, postformal thought-based roles might permit greater creativity in using strategies to solve problems where the problem goal is unclear. Most everyday problems fall into this category.

Systems theory and adult sex roles: Systems theory is a theory of interacting processes and the way they influence each other over time to permit the continuity of some larger whole. Systems act so as to continue. Systems change because their own balances are not optimal or because they are influenced by other systems. Some authors who provide excellent descriptions of these general ideas are van Bertalanffy and Miller. Miller's discussion of living systems is especially useful to consider for a discussion of sex roles. Individuals, societies, and cells all appear to use similar processes to create boundaries, to take in stimulation, to process information, to act, and to change. For example, for cells, information may be chemical and may be filtered by cell walls; for persons, information may be conceptual and may be filtered by perceptions; for societies information may be news and be filtered by censors. Cells, persons, and societies all exist in relation to each other which further complicates matters. Within systems theory, roles are structures of the social system which are equivalent to organs in the physical/person system;

they are organized ways of ensuring that some vital function is performed.

As living systems—be they cell, person, or society- develop and age, they appear to proceed through a regular set of stages. They begin in disorder, that is, with a few parts concrete and defined. They become more orderly, defined, and bounded over time. They become rigid before they disintegrate and die as systems. System changes may be further described in chaos theory and complexity theory.

How does this relate to sex role development over the life span? Consider the person and society as living systems, each seeking continuity and meeting survival needs. These needs include control of information and energy flow. Sex roles are ways person and social systems can regulate the flow of information and energy (effort) while taking care of survival needs. The early stages of these systems are disordered in regard to roles, i.e., no roles are apparent. For example, the newborn in sex roleless, and a group of strangers is roleless as a group. Later stages are associated with more concretized roles; in the person and in the group, masculinity and femininity may emerge. Final stages find the roles rigid and inflexible, so they would fail to respond to the pull of new needs. This failure of response leads to disorder and a search of new, more complex order. Systems theory suggests that this may be the kind of transition we are seeing in societies now, and in the individual after the reproductive period and parental imperative (Gutmann). The person having rigid roles (sex roles or other roles), faced with new demands, might adapt with new complex integrations of role related behaviours, or might keep a dysfunctional system.

Sex role research: Six major conflicts have emerged in the field. Future research is likely to focus on these, as well as moving along to others. First, are roles fixed or flexible? Early theorists saw roles as fixed, at an early age, for life. More recent theorists see roles established, then evolving, based on age, societal demands, etc. Second, how central are roles to personality? In more traditional societies sex roles seem to be a core organizing principle of personal functioning; in less traditional cultures, they seem to be adopted and cast off with less impact on the peron's sense of self. Third, how closely do roles relate to identity? This is a subdivision of the second question. Fourth, should roles be measured taking into account context and self-perception us actual behavior? If roles need not be fixed, context might be extremely important to self-description since success as a parent (for example) often requires different traits than success as an employee. In another example, the single female parent may best use a combined role the earlier theorists labeled "masculine" as well as "feminine." Also, one's consistent self-concept, as perceived by the self, may be very different from what witnesses see the person actually doing, since the person may be verbally expressing what he or she has been told should be said. Fifth, are stereotypes, sexism, and power politics inherent in sex roles? Some theorists maintain that since roles have always been connected to power, domination, discrimination, and stereotypes, that this is a part of their dynamics. Consideration of these conflicts, and the issues on which theorists agree, leads to several recommendations for future research and theory. Several conclusions can be drawn from the early and the recent literature on life span sex role development.

1. We must not jump to conclusions that responses on a scale will be predictive of behavior. Individuals may say that they are "masculine" by their scale responses, but may mean they are masculine in regard to stereotyping concepts. They may rate themselves differently in other situations, may act other than their ratings, and their behaviour may vary from situation to situation. They may do what is most rewarding and that may happen to be masculine. They may score themselves masculine due to development of an identity labeled masculine. They may do so since masculine behavior is socially desirable. They may change in self-definition due to life stage demands, or when their own concept of masculinity is no longer like their behaviour, even if to everyone else they are still "masculine," by some other definition. And they may lable themselves or act as they perceive society excepts them to do. Since all these factors may underlie their responses to the scale, it is hard to predict behaviour based on scale responses.

2. Responses to sex role instruments do mean something. What is meant may be tempered by each perons's perception of unspoken situational constraints and other factors mentioned above. If individuals respond appropriately they are matching themselves to global standards designed to reflect the clearest opposition between gender-assigned roles.

3. Masculinity, feminity, and androgyny have been shown to be adaptive. Depending upon the situational demands, subject to the constraints above, any of the roles might be adaptive. The real question is, what is the most useful role in a certain setting; masculine, feminine, both, or

neither? Useful may mean "liable to be rewarded" or "consistent", or "workable by some external criterion." Androgyny may be the most adaptive response in terms of the last criterion; masculinity may be the most adaptive in terms of the first.

4. Sex roles are meaningful in terms of social expectations. The concept of global, oppositional, gender-linked roles is present for all members of society, and society imposes these role expectations on individuals so long as the real characteristics of those individuals are not known. So whatever complex designation of role and behaviour one adopts, the general "other" is still seen as conforming to the global stereotypes. Individuals also perceive role expectations projected by others, and, to the degree they are conformists, attempt to conform to them.

5. Sex roles are meaningful ways to order one's sense of self as socially efficacious, to create a sense of personal conformity, and to order self-concept. The creation of the self concept is partially accomplished by acting, and noticing that the self is the center of effective acts. Roles permit structured action likely to work in a society. They also are labels that live on beyond the individual and can be generalized to many situations. Knowing a sex role without knowing the meaning of that role to the person is to take only half a step toward knowledge.

6. The meaning of sex roles depends on age and developmental stage. Meanings are related to modes of cognition and social demands at each period. They are also related to the previous history and experience of the person and the historical period in which the society finds itself. Infants can

know roles in direct physical forms, but cannot know them abstractly. The concrete operational person can know roles in the abstract, and the formal operational person can build logical systems of roles. The postformal person can see roles relativistically, as co-created by persons in them.

7. Models of sex role changes over time can be of many types. Change can be more complex than increase or decrease in global qualities. Change might occur on one dimension but not on another, or in global role traits but not in behaviour, or visa versa. Change might be triggered by specific events or might represent an accretion over time. It may be reversible. Change might result from diffusion of a self-concept until its meaning is so muddy that it can become something new. Change might depend on past rates of change. It is useful for investigators to be clear about their underlying model of change as they discuss sex role development.

8. Sex role complexity and adult sex role development may be linked to cognitive abilities like postformal thought or problem-solving skills. Roles have been linked to cognitive processes such as concept formation. As cognitive operations become more complex, their associated roles might be seen as multifaceted rather than undimensional.

9. Sex role development related questions (e.g., "Am I being feminine?" "What is the masculine thing to do at any age?") may be conceptualized in decision theory or problem solving theory as ill-structured problems. This means among other things that they have an unclear goal. Decisions must be made about the nature of the goal as a part of solving the problem. Problem-solving

literature can be a guide to dimensions we need to test to understand the process of solving sex role behaviour/self-concept problems. This application of cognitive theory has not yet been attempted.

10. Sex role developmental theories suggest new physics concepts and might make use of them. A multivariate approach needs to be taken in sex role studies, in that adjacent centers of causality—other persons, the social order—cause changes in an individual's sex roles. The person, in turn, causes changes in the social order by his or her perception of roles and by action on that perception. It is clear that one's vantage point in measuring sex roles is very important in drawing conclusions about the results. These models have companion models in the physical sciences that could be used in studies of change, both change in a person and change among systems.

11. Sex role development theory can make use of ideas in systems theory. Personal and social systems are connected by many roles, among them sex roles. Theories of living systems give us an outline of the processes within and between those two systems. The flow of information can be studied within and between systems and roles are part of that information flow. A study of system boundaries can be conceptualized as a study of rigid or flexible roles and the capability of society or person to perceive or enact them. Future studies can take this model of living systems into account. Models of complexity and chaos may also be useful.

12. Emerging ideas suggest that in the future roles will be orchestrated consciously by the person, rather than being imposed consciously or unconsciously by society, or being left to the mercy

of unexamined forces. Each child may grow up aware that she or he has a wide spectrum of role possibilities that can be acted out.

Homosexuality: Sexual orientation, as it relates to homosexuality, is one's erotic attraction toward the same sex. Sexual orientation is a part of one's sexual identity, which, in turn, is primarily related to physical and emotional disposition, and is simultaneously interconnected yet distinct from biological and gender identity.

In Western culture, the most prominent means of conceptualizing sexual orientation is in terms of hetero-versus homosexuality. Traditionally, such distinctions are oversimplified and create oppositional positions. For these reasons, some theorists would rather conceive of orientation as being on a continuum, with heterosexuality and homosexuality at either end and in between a vast gradation of overlap reflecting bisexuality. Dichotomous thinking, coupled with rigid cultural values biased in in favor of the heterosexual majority have led to a lengthy history of intolerance towards and oppression of homosexual and bisexual individuals.

Two forces helped shape negative and oppressive attitudes toward homosexuality. The first was Judeo—Christian values and beliefs that held that nonprocreative sexual acts were regarded as "sins again nature" and consequently frowned on in the culture. The second force was the rise of medicine and psychology as powerful authorities and arbiters of social morality by defining and controlling "deviant" and "diseased" behaviours. This control led to the condemnation of many fringe or nontraditional sexual practice with homosexuality in the forefront. Psychiatry, for example, included homosexuality in their diagnostic manual thus sanctioning intervention and treatment. Sin was now replaced by pathology. Being identified as mentally ill meant that homosexuals could be stripped of their civil and human rights while the heterosexual population looked on.

Under fire from within and outside their ranks, on December 15,1973, the American Psychiatric Association board of trustees voted to remove homosexuality from the categories of mental illness. After much struggle and debate, homosexuality was replaced with a new category, ego-dystonic homosexuality, denoting those homosexual individuals who were distressed by their orientation and wanted to become heterosexual. This compromise category did not last for long, as many professionals and lay persons could see that it was just another more subtle means of perpetuating prejudice and oppression. Finally, all reference to homosexuality was removed from the official nomenclature and the following excerpt was inserted in the DSM-II-R:

This category [ego-dystonic] has been eliminated fors several reasons. It suggested to some that homosexuality itself was considered a disorder. In the United States almost all people who are homosexual first go through a phse in which their homosexuality is ego-dystonic. Furthermore, the diagnosis of ego-dystonic homosexuality has rarely been used clinically and there have been only a few articles in the scientific literature that use the concept.

Prevalence: The problem in measuring the prevalence of homosexuality is that it must be operationally defined. Renowned sex reseacher Alfred Kinsey chose to operationally define sexual orientation on a continuum in terms of behaviour frequency of homo-, hetero-, and degree of combined sexual behaviours.

To conceive of homosexuality in strict behavioural terms challenged the more prevalent practice of using the terms to represent a personality deficit. The latter approach, of course, leads to social stigmatization Kinsey also avoided applying sexual orientation labels in an either/or manner, by conceiving of sexuality as a range of behaviours on a continuum. Despite his popularity, his results were criticized on methodological and theoretical grounds. Specifically, grave doubts were raised about the generalizability of his data from the limited sampling he used. Other researchers conducting surveys with better sampling methods found similar to much lesser rates of incidence; usually between 4 and 16% homosexual behaviour of some kinds. Theoretically, Kinsey was critized for being too reductionistic by trying to conceptualize the homosexual experience in terms of the frequency of same sex behaviours. Regardless of the precise percentages and how one exactly conceives of it, homosexuality is and has been a pervasive part of our culture and population.

Since the early 1970s, there appears to have been a radical rethinking of how we treat those of homo-or bisexual orientations. Still, some lay persons and professionals find these orientations pathological and must seek causes and roots for these disorders. Katchadourian responds to these efforts in the following manner.

Those who accept homosexuality as an illness

seek its causes. Those who do not, object to this approach. "Causes" implies that there is something wrong; why not seek the "causes" of heterosexuality? The search for the origins of sexual orientation—homosexual or heterosexual—is a more legitimate quest.

The causal agents responsible for producing any sexual orientation are basically unknown. If we hope to gain insight by relying on a single explanation, then we will surely miss the dynamic and interactive nature of sexual identity. Whether the theoretical model is based upon genetic inheritance, developmental influences, or psychodynamic conflict, the nature of sexual orientation, regardless of sexual preference, seems better understood as having multiple roots.

Treatments: Contemporary though rejects the outdated notion of homosexuality and bisexuality as diseases to be treated and cured. Attempts by professionals to change or convert homosexuals into heterosexuals have almost always been exercises in futility. Despite long and intensive therapeutic hours, psycho-analysis has had no success. With their aversive counter—conditioning techniques, the behavioural therapies have only faired marginally better. Irrespective of the theoretical model, when a person (homosexual or not) is forced into the therapy room, not only is change highly unlikely bust the chances for negative psychological consequences are greatly increased.

An apparent exception to this lack of success was the Master and Johnson sex therapy study, which reported to have "helped" two-thirds of those who volunteered for a 2-week treatment program.

Criticisms of their work include the fact that the male and female participants were carefully screened to ensure that they exhibited high levels of desire to change and were the beneficiaries of very supportive partners. In addition to such biases in sampling, further analysis of the follow-up data revealed that the claimed failure rate of only 28% was probably too low. Perhaps a rate of about 45% would be more accurate.

Differences in health and personality: As pointed out earlier, psychiatrists have conceptualized the homosexual as inherently pathological and heterosexual as "normal." Numerous scientific studies have compared homosexuals who sought treatment against-nornal heterosexuals who were not in treatment. Differences were found between these groups on health and personality variables. More recent studies, with improved methodology, have shown that very few differences in pathology actually exist between equivalent heterosexual and homosexual samples. Differences in depression and suicide rates previously attributed to pathology or flaws in the individuals are now seen from a broader socio-psychological level of causation, i.e., environmental pressures to live up to one's societal status as deviant.

Another area in which scientific bias has played a mystifying role is in the realm of personality differences between homo-and heterosexuals. Specifically, there have been studies showing gay men were more feminine than straight men and that lesbians were more masculine than their heterosexual counterparts. Once again, such findings have been shown to be based on methodologically flawed clinical/non-clinical designs. Once corrected for biased sampling, such studies show that the differences in gender identity are minimal. Yes, "butch" lesbians and effeminate gays exist, but as a stereotype they are not representative of the homosexual and bisexual population as a whole.

The direct assessment of the genital aspect of sexual behaviour in all three response systems presents every possible roadblock to behavioural assessment. This behaviour ordinarily occurs in places remote from the therapeutic setting. Because of the very nature of sexual behaviour, these places are most often those that cannot be directly observed or monitored to allow the proper assessment. Indeed, the cultural sanctions against attempting any such assessment would ensure that, if they were carried out on a wide scale, the behaviour would be so altered as to bear little resemblance to it normal and usual occurrence. Ordinarily, when behaviour cannot be observed in the natural environment, contrived situations are constructed to assess the nature and strength of a given behaviour in a more convenient setting. But the sensitivity of sexual behaviour in our culture makes assessment of the full range of sexual behaviour, even in a contrived laboratory situation, extremely difficult. It is to the credit of Masters and Johnson that the cultural restrictions against the direct assessment of sexual responding in a laboratory situation were broken. Through this research the physichological mechanisms of the genital aspects of human sexual behaviour were clarified, paving the way for a more careful and valid assessment of various aspects of the chain of behaviours making up the human sexual response. Since most investigators and clinicians lack the facilities and/or the administrative and community support to study the end points of genital sexual behaviour, such as heterosexual intercourse, alternative procedures have been developed. These procedures have in common a movement back down the behavioural chain to a point where earlier aspects of sexual arousal and measured. The assumption has been that sexual arousal is a necessary step in the chain leading to the consummation of sexual behaviour. As such, changes in the strength or patterns of sexual arousal will have a direct relation to the strength or patterns of later behaviours in the chain.

There are other reasons why assessment of early components of the chain are desirable. For instance, in certain sexual deviations such as pedophilia, a patient may be able to engage in adult heterosexual intercourse on repeated occasions. A more careful examination of his behavioural chain however, will reveal he is accomplishing this by engaging in those behaviros that ordinarily would lead to a pedophilic interchange. The most important of these behaviours will be intense pedophilic fantasies that will continue through intercourse. Some patients are able to carry on their behaviour over a period of years although they report the act of intercourse itself to be aversive. If satisfying hetero-sexual relationships are the goal, then events that precede intercourse, such as interest in social behaviours and sexual features of the partner, as well as fantasies of heterosexual interactions, are important targets for assessment and treatment. In view of these relationships, assessment of early events in the chain of the genital aspects of sexual behaviour may be more important to long-lasting sexual satisfaction than assessment of the end point of this chain. A second reason for assessing early components in the chain is a practical one. Many patients with sexual problems do not have a partner with whom they can interact sexually. Measures requiring such interaction would then not be possible. These factors notwithstanding, one must be careful not to over interpret data based on assessment of sexual arousal. The assumption has been made over the years that arousal is a necessary precursor to later genital behaviour. the example of the married pedophiliac illustrates, however, that arousal patterns often are not absolutely necessary for later consummation behaviour. Bancroft noted as early as 1971 that arousal itself bears an uncertain relationship to later sexual behavior. The large role played by conginitive representations of sexual stimuli and the effect of these representations on arousal patterns led Bancroft to suggest that both sexual behaviour and arousal patterns should be assessed whenever possible.

More recently, Caird and Wincze observed that the correlation between sexual arousal and other aspects of sexual behaviour in women may also be poor at times. In their clinical experience they have observed women complaining of deficiencies in sexual arousal who report orgasm rates as high a 75 per cent during intercourse. They also report women who have normal levels of arousal and who even initiate sexual contacts at a high frequency, yet who rarely if ever experience orgasm.

Yet another problem with objective measures of sexual arousal is that they occur in contrived situations, and the relationship between sexual arousal measured in the laboratory and later sexual behaviour outside the laboratory is uncertain. It is also true that the relationship between sexual arousal in a contrived laboratory situation and sexual arousal in the patient's natural environment is not clear. Even the relationship between sexual arousal in the laboratory and sexual behaviour in a similar contrived laboratory situation is unknown. The popularity in clinical settings of assessing sexual arousal in contrived situations, then, is based on its high discriminate validity when compared to other psychophysiological measures of arousal and also on a high correlation with what reliable people report their sexual arousal patterns and behaviour in the natural environment to be. One clear goal is the development of procedures to assess sexual behaviour as well as sexual arousal in contrived situations. A first step might be the creation of situations in the laboratory when at least the initial stages of approach and contact can be recreated and observed. Forgione has recently used mannikins of children to assess approach behaviour in pedophiliacs. He reports that while approaching and fondling the mannikins these patients engage in a variety of behaviours not reported in a detailed interview.

Similarly, Marks, Gelder, and Bancroft allowed transvestites to cross-dress in a contrived laboratory setting as part of treatment. However, there is no reason why this could not be a behavioural assessment procedure independent of treatment. In assessing heterosocial skills, this type of contrived situation is common.

A more remote but equally important goal would be the development of methods to observe approach behaviour in the natural environment. The practical and ethical problems inherent in this type of assessment seem overwhelming at the present time, but in view of advances in naturalistic observation and the relaxation of attitudes toward sexual behaviour in our society, something like this may be possible, assuming the ethical issue could be resolved. The increased use of female collaborators in clinical treatment of sexual problems could possibly be extended to naturalistic studies of sexual approach behaviour in males and similar, procedures could be used to assess behaviours leading up to genital interactions in females.

The early success in establishing certain types of validity for objective measures of early components in the chain of sexual behaviour, such as sexual arousal, has led to an exaggerated idea of the usefulness of these measures, but used and interpreted properly, these measures are essential in a complete assessment of sexual behaviour. Procedures most useful in the assessment of components of early sexual arousal measure both physiological and self-report aspects in both the male and female. Physiological measures of early male sexual arousal, specifically erections, have been available longer than measures of female arousal and have been subjected to wider experimentation and validation.

Objective measurement of male sexual arousal: A recent view article by Zuckerman was largely responsible for the upsurge in interest in measurement of male erections. Until the publication of this review, penile erection was but one of many physiological measures employed in the assessment of sexual arousal. Other measures, such as GRS, cardiac rate, respiration, and pupil size, were thought to be valid and reliable indicators of sexual arousal. Although changes in these responses do occur during sexual arousal, Zuckerman concluded from his review that other emotional states, such as fear, anger, and pain, could cause similar changes. The nonspecificity or lack of discriminate validity obviated the usefulness of these measures. Penile erections, however, were specific to sexual arousal with the exception of rare, pathological physical conditions. These conclusions renewed interest in devices and procedures to measure erections and caused a flurry of activity devoted to investigating the relative merits of existing apparatus.

The increased interest in arousal and erections during the late 1960s and the 1970s in turn activated the psychohistorians, who wondered if interest in erections was a modern phenomenon or something also of interest to our forefathers (foremothers?). In their search the historians once again discovered that very little is new in the world and that farmers at the turn of the century were concerned about excessive masturbation by their horses. In addition to being unsightly, and perhaps immoral, this practice resulted in a low sperm count and an inability to impregnate mares. To prevent it they built a large, cuff-like apparatus that enclosed the horse's penis and testicles. The beginnings of tumesence of the penis connected two points which then set off an alarm connected to the device. The inventor of the device noted that when the alarm rang, the horse needed some attention. Some modern-day theorists might say, however, that the alarm was effective because it interrupted the horse's sexual fantasies.

In Czechoslovakia in the late 1950s Kurt Freund developed an apparatus that would quantify erectile responses. He was also the first to use the apparatus in any serious manner in sex research. The development of this device, which is still in use, was a major advance in the measurement of male sexual behaviour. Essentially, Freund's apparatus is a glass cylinder with a rubber cuff on one end into which the penis is inserted. As the penis enlarges, the amount of air displaced in the cylinder is measured. Thus this device measures penile volume changes. In reviewing various apparatuses to quantify penile erections, Able and Blanchard have described a variety of such devices. Jovanovic had published a similar review earlier. At the present time, however, all devices can be classified into two categories—those that measure penile volume and those that quantify penile circumference changes.

Freund and his colleagues described his device to measure penile volume in a technical article in 1965. Freund has utilized his apparatus in numerous investigations over the year and continues to collect data important to the field of sex research has also developed a volumetric device that is somewhat simpler and less expensive.

More recently, two devices have been developed to measure penile circumference changes. The first utilizes mercury-filled tubing. Bancroft, Jones, and Pullan devised an apparatus that was similar to one described by Fisher, Gross, and Zuch. Essentially this apparatus was a mercury-filled elastic tube that encircled the penis. As penile tumesence occurred, the elastic tube lengthened around the penis causing contraction of the inner diameter of the tubing. In Bancroft's device, which has been adopted by a number of researchers, the mercury-filled tubing forms one arm of a

Wheatstone bridge circuit. As tumesence occurs and the diameter of the mercury in the tubing decreases, electrical resistance of the mercury column is increased. The electrical changes can then be recorded. Bancroft described the technology of this device in some detail.

A second widely used device to measure penile circumference was developed by Barlow, Becker, Leitenberg, and Agras. It is a thin, metal, ring-like device open at one end that is placed around the penis, forming a semicircle around it. At the base of the ring are located one or more strain gauges. During erection, the "wings" of the ring separate, which causes a slight bending of the strain gauge and produces increased electrical output. The device is easily calibrated by fashioning a smooth wooden cone on which the full range of circumferences is indicated by a pencil. For calibration, one simply runs the ring up and down the cone noting the read-out at the penciled size indicators. This process demonstrates a remarkably linear output over the full range of circumference changes that is stable over time.

No formal comparison of the mercury tubing or strain gauge methods of measuring-penile circumference has yet been undertaken, although informal comparisons in our laboratory indicate that the strain gauge produces a more linear output over a wider range of cylindrical sizes when calibrated on wooden cones. In addition, owing to its design, the strain gauge device is more rugged than the mercury tubing in that it is less susceptible to damage. Furthermore, the mercury gauge is expandable over only 10 percent of its resting length and tends to separate at the upper range of displacement regardless of the size of the tube's boring. The mercury gauge has also been reported as restrictive. Because there is no restriction of expansion, the strain gauge requires six times less force than the mercury gauge to achieve the same amount of expansion. Further aspects of train gauge technology can be found in Barlow et al. A disadvantage of the strain gauge device, when compared to the mercury tubing, is cost. The strain gauge currently costs in the neighbourhood of $25.00 to $50.00 as compared to $5.00 to $10.00 for the mercury tubing, although the recent initiation of commercial production of the strain gauge device may lower the cost somewhat.

In reviewing the two devices Bancroft notes that the strain gauge devices may be more prone to movement artifacts. In our experience movement artifacts have not been a problem and when they do occur, they are easily identifiable on any read-out. Nevertheless, none of these comments represent data, and all subjective impressions are easily testable. When they are properly used, it would seem that the devices would be equally satisfactory, with the strain gauge possessing a slight advantage based on durability, ease of handling and less restrictiveness.

Comparison of volumetric and circumferential devices: Several investigators have recently directly compared circumferential devices with volumetric devices. In Freund's laboratory in Toronto the Barlow et al. strain gauge was compared with Freund's original volume device. Volunteer subjects wore both devices while exposed to erotic stimulation. Independently, McConaghy in Australia also compared volumetric versus circumferential devices, in this case the mercury tubing device.

Although the data were complex, the general conclusion was that volumetric devices are more sensitive and pick up changes at smaller penile sizes than circumference devices. Although both devices are capable of picking up low levels of arousal of which the patient is often unaware, the volume devices are usually employed in studies where measurement of low levels of arousal are necessary. Circumferential devices, on the other hand, are more flexible and less cumbersome and are usually employed in studies measuring larger, more functional levels of arousal, in the range of 25 to 100 percent of a full erection.

The relative complexity of a device to measure volume versus circumference contributes to two other differences between the two approaches Volumetric devices are considerably more expensive, and enclosing the entire penis as they do, they are more cumbersome an difficult to work with than the circumferential devices that are quite easily positioned by the subject himself. Nevertheless, these difference are probably not important because the trend in assessment of sexual arousal is to choose a specific measurement device, basing one's choice on the purpose of the study. Because volumetric devices are more sensitive and pick up smaller changes, the apparatus has often been used in theoretical studies of patterns of sexual arousal when large amounts of arousal are not necessary to test certain hypotheses. For example, Freund, Langevin, Cibiri, and Zajac demonstrated that homosexuals showed no more detumescence to heterosexual slides than heterosexuals to homosexual slides. The purpose of the experiment was to text the theory that homosexuals have a hetero-sexual phobia.

Absolute amounts of arousal were not necessary to test this hypothesis. A second common use of volume devices is diagnosis or assessment of various arousal patterns in individuals or groups. The sensitivity of the volumetric device will allow the pin-pointing of patterns of arousal, even if individuals are instructed to mask or suppress the arousal.

Circumferential measures, on the other hand, being less cumbersome, more sturdy, and relatively less expensive, are effective in measuring the large, functionally relevant levels of sexual arousal useful in assessing changes in patterns or levels of arousal as a result of treatment. The goals here are quite different. Sexual arousal less than 20 percent of a full erection may have decided theoretical interest but be of little or no clinical value to the patient attempting to learn a new functional pattern of arousal. More arousal, in the area of 75 percent of a full erection, is necessary. This may account for the differential methods of reporting data obtained from volume versus circumferential devices. Volumetric devices often report data in terms of scores, rank order scores, or other methods to make the data more amenable to statistical analysis. The disadvantage of this method, of course, is that one is unable to determine the quantity or range of arousal with which the investigation is working. Circumferential measures, on the other hand, most often report data in terms of a percentage of full erection. Although this method is-less sensitive to statistical comparisons, the clinical implications of the arousal with which one is working are readily apparent.

This discussion implies a growing specificity of function for volumetric and circumferential devices, but it would be premature to draw conclusions on the optimal uses of these devices at this time. Circumferential devices, although somewhat less sensitive, have been used successfully to study low levels of arousal and to assess diagnostic or more theoretical questions. Conversely, there is obvious reason why volumetric devices could not be used to measure larger erctions, as in the assessment of change during treatment. Considerably more data are needed in this important area of assessment.

Objective measurement of female sexual arousal: The study of female sexual arousal has lagged behind that of male sexual arousal as scientists in the field have awaited the development of the proper technology. Despite the demonstrated nonspecificity of general physiological measures, nothing else has been available, and some investigators have conducted investigations using multiple physiological measures. The most exciting development in sex research in the past dead has been the development of a vaginal photo-plethysmograph, which is a measure of female sexual arousal having the same discriminate validity as erection measures in males. Based on the pioneering work of Masters an Johnson, this device was constructed to take advantage of the massive, localized vasocongestive reaction that occurs in the vaginal wall early in sexual arousal. Essentially, the probe measures the amount of light reflected from vaginal wall tissue. The less light reflected, the more vasocongestion and, hence, the more arousal. Geer et al. originally validated this device as a measure of sexual arousal.

More recently, Hoon, Wincze, and Hoon have developed and described what seems to be an improved probe device, which substitutes an infrared light source and a phototransistor detector cell that may eliminate artifacts in the original device. Although the improvements seem logical, they have yet to be demonstrated as being more efficient. Moe important, the two devices work on exactly the same principle, and some preliminary date on validity are available. In a model study Hoon, Wincze, and Hoon demonstrated that the infrared photoplethys-mograph measures blood volume changes and not changes mediated by veginal wall contractions or changes in lubrication. In a second important experiment, designed to determine whether the device discriminates sexual arousal from other arousal states. Hoon et al. illustrated clear differences between sexually arousing, dysphoric, and neutral emotional conditions in women. Systolic blood pressure discriminated normal from sxeually dysfunctional women, but other physiological indicators, such as heartrate, did not. Hoon et al. are already beginning to employ this device to assess changes during treatment of sexual problems in women in the same way measures of erection are used in assessment of male sexual problems. In Geer's laboratory Heiman also found that arousal measured by the probe device was less for anorgasmic women viewing erotic films than for orgasmic women, and recently Geer and Quartararo have demonstrated that measurement of changes in vaginal blood volume provides in some women an unambiguous indication of orgasm.

Although the probe device is in use in only a few laboratories at this time, the early data are extremely promising. In addition, the ease of handling and use should ensure a rapid expansion of research on female sexual arousal.

Stimulus modalities, content, and methods in the objective measurement of sexual arousal: With the advent of valid devices for the assessment of sexual arousal, investigators have worked on refining their procedures so as to assess a variety of arousal patterns under optimal conditions. One of the first questions that occurred to various investigators when they were measuring male sexual arousal was: What is the optimal stimulus modality that will set the occasion for the greatest amounts of arousal? Investigators and clinicians have used movies, videotapes, slides, and free fantasies, as well as the audiotape method mentioned earlier. In one recent experiment modalities of stimuli were compared in people with different patterns of arousal. A group of 20 voluntary homosexual subjects were presented with a two-minute clip of videotapes depicting homosexual interactions, the audiotapes describing the same homosexual interactions, or slides. These three stimuli were presented twice in each of three successive sessions, for a total of six stimuli per session, in random order. During the first session, subjects were told to become involved with the person described or depicted. In the second session they were also told to become involved but to suppress their erection response by any mental mens. In the third session they were once again told to involve themselves with the person in the situation. The results indicated that the videotape produced the largest amount of arousal, even when subjects were attempting to suppress this arousal. Slides produced an intermediate level of arousal. Some suppression of arousal occurred during both moveies and slides. It is interesting to note that audiotapes produced the least arousal; however, subjects seemed unable to suppress this arousal when asked to do so. Other studies indicate that he general pattern in which movies or videotapes produce maximal arousal is also true for heterosexuals and exhibitionists. However, for more idiosyncratic patterns of arousal, or patterns that are more difficult to represent of film, such as pedophilia, audiotapes would seem the preferred method . Movies, audiotapes, and fantasies have also been used with success to occasion sexual arousal in females, but no comparison of these modalities has been reported.

Yet another question concerns the structure of heterosexual arousal. In behavioural assessment there are often criterion behaviours decided on by the patient and the therapist that then become the goal of behavioural intervention. It is difficult to determine the criterion behaviours, however, if one is not aware of the population norms for a given set of behaviours. in assessment of sexual arousal it was assumed for a period that an explicit film depicting heterosexual intercourse, which elicited arousal in heterosexuals, would not elicit arousal in people with other patterns of arousal. This proved not to be true. For instance, homosexuals look at this complex stimuli, focus on the male in the scene, and become quite aroused. Transexuals look at the same stimuli and become aroused for quite a different reason; they identify with the female in the scene and fantasize that they are making love to the male. Thus it is important in assessment to develop content that discriminates one group from another so as to provide meaningful and valid assessment of changes during any intervention.

To determine the stimulus content that discriminates heterosexuals from people with other patterns of arousal, six volunteer exclusive heterosexuals and six volunteer exclusive homosepuals were shown four videotapes with different content in the study by Mavissakalisn et al. One videotape depicted a nude woman assuming various sexual postures. A second depicted a lesbian couple engaged in lovemaking. A third depicted a heterosexual couple engaged in sexual intercourse. The fourth depicted a male homosexual couple engaged in lovemaking. Over the course of two sessions, each subject saw examples of each content area four times, for a total of sixteen video clips that were counterbalanced for content. Penile circumference changes were measured along with subjective reports of arousal and reports on a pleasantness- unpleasantness continuum for each film clip.

It is clear from these data, which are presented in terms of average penile circumference change based on percentage of full erection as well as average rate of arousal and on a zero to 100 scale, that the heterosexual film clip did not discriminate beteen homosexual and heterosexual subjects. Even the single girl did not discriminate these groups although there was a trend in that direction. The two film clips that clearly discriminated the two groups were the lesbian couple and the male homosexual couple. Heterosexuals responded with significantly more arousal to the lesbian couple than did homosexuals, and the reverse was true for the homosexual film clip. These data indicate that arousal to lesbian films should be the criterion when one is attempting to instigate heterosexual arousal.

Sandford has also analyzed the structure of heterosexual arousal. He measured erection responses to films of women engaging in various sexually oriented behaviours as well as to films of couples engaging in sexual behaviours. A woman alone, either stripping of naked, produced less arousal than depictions of intercourse in various positions. Geer has begun a major research project whose purpose is to determine culturally prescribed modal patterns of sexual arousal, based on Gagnon's social scripting theory of sexuality. If these investigators can determine a sequence of sexual behaviour to which arousal increased in a linear fashion, these patterns will then become "criterion" patterns for use in individual assessment. Preliminary efforts with audiotapes indicate that this is feasible and, furthermore, that male and female sexual arousal correlate highly to an audiotaped sequence of sexually related events or behaviours.

In one of the more sophisticated and detailed investigations on the structure of sexual arousal, Freund, McKnight,Langevin, and Cibiri investigated sexual arousal patterns of adult heterosexual males along several continuua. Stimulus slides and moving pictures of males and females of various ages, some as young as six to eight years old, were shown to 40 adult males. In addition, different parts of the anatomy in each of the various age groups were selected to determine the specificity of sexual arousal. The results indicated that heterosexual adults respond not only to adult women but also to girls as young as eight years old, with the public and chest areas being the most erotic.

One valid method of investigating sexual arousal patterns therefore, is to show erotic material in various stimulus modalities for brief periods to large groups of people. Average responses are calculated to determine modal response patterns. A second equally valid approach uses variation of withdrawal designs in single-case methodology. In this approach sexual arousal is measured repeatedly as erotic stimuli in various modalities are introduced and withdrawn. This method is illustrated by procedures used in the assessment of a foot fetish described earlier. This method is also illustrated in some interesting recent attempts to assess the sexual arousal of rapists. The use of the repeated presentation of erotic stimuli to assess changes during treatment for sexual arousal patterns has been in use for some time.

The relation of cognitive factors to sexual arousal: In 1972 Zuckerman, in a presentation at the American Psychological Association, posed the question, "Does the penis lie? "His conclusion was, yes, the penis can lie if the mind distracts or deludes its owner. Zuckerman's paper was a statement on the relation of cognitive activity to patterns of sexual arousal . This aspect of the physiological assessment of sexual arousal patterns, is one that most sex researchers would like to ignore. The fact is that subjects can suppress erections during periods of sexual arousal. Geer has confirmed Zuckerman's supposition that "distraction" may lead to suppression. In a clever experiment Geer demonstrated through the use of a dichotic listening paradigm that erotic descriptions presented in one ear of the subject were highly arousing but produced erections only when a cognitive task presented in the other ear, to which the subject was required to attend, was not complex. As the cognitive task became more complex, erections diminished. In analogue laboratory experiment using heterosexual volunteers Laws and Rubin and Henson and Rubin investigated subjects' ability to suppress erections while watching erotic films. Even while subjects were describing the particular film they were viewing, they could suppress their erections if instructed to do so. Able et al. demonstrated that a group of subjects with homosexual arousal patterns could also suppress erections. However, the ability of subjects in the Henson and Rubin experiment to suppress erections while watching and verbalizing the content of the film, suggests that further experimental analysis is necessary to isolate the factors involved. These experiments do illustrate, however, the importance of cognitive activity in patterns of sexual arousal and sexual behaviour.

The implication of this work is that assessment of arousal patterns may have little relation to the measurement of arousal or sexual behaviour beyond the limitations to external validity. Using clinical populations, Freund examined this issue by asking both homosexuals and heterosexuals to attempt to hide their arousal patterns and fake alternative arousal patterns. Only a few subjects were actually able to fake their arousal patterns, using Freund's sensitive assessment of volume. Under slightly different conditions, only five out of 42 heterosexuals and six out of 24 homosexuals were successful at faking their arousal patterns. in a later study only one out of 27 pedophiliacs was able to represent himself as exclusively heterosexual for adult women. Although several more were able to fake a heterosexual arousal pattern, only one was able to hide his pedophiliac pattern of arousal completely. In line with these more encouraging findings, it should be noted that subjects in the Henson and Rubin study still averaged measurable arousal even under instructions to suppress arousal. Similarly, homosexual subjects in the Abel *et al.* study did not suppress below 20 percent of a full erection on the average. This is certainly enough for adequate assessment, particularly if one is using the more sensitive volumetric devices. Whether one would attempt to assess patterns of arousal against the subject's wishes is, of course, an ethical issues.

Nevertheless, the fact is that subjects or patients can suppress sexual arousal, and this fact must be taken into consideration during any assessment of patterns of sexual. To facilitate arousal and circumvent suppression for whatever reasons, one should use the strongest erotic stimuli possible and arrange the laboratory situation to facilitate attention to the erotic stimulus. These studies illustrate the importance of cognitive activity and demonstrate again the importance of collecting attitudinal and self-report measures in a comprehensive assessment of sexual arousal behaviour. The next section reviews and discusses the variety of assessment techniques and procedures subsumed under the category of self-report.

Assessment of sexual arousal behaviour by self-report: The preceding section described procedures for the physiological assessment of sexual arousal. With the few exceptions cited, there has been no important work on the development of direct behavioural observations of sexual arousal or behaviour. However, as one might expect, the third response system, self-report, has undergone considerable development because it was the only method available to sex researchers for several years.

We noted earlier that self- report measures of sexual arousal and behaviour can be broken down into several distinct entities. Unfortunately, there is little agreement in the field of psychological assessment on the nature of content of these entities. Following the categories of Whalen, Bacroft mentions at least four categories: (1) sexual preferences and other sexual attitudes; (2) sexual gratification (i.e., the mutuality and intensity of sexual pleasure); (3) sexual arousability (i.e., the capacity to respond to sexual stimulation with increased sexual arousal); and (4) sexual activity, fantasized or real. Quinn, Graham, Harbison, and McAllister suggest three categories; (1) sexual orientation that attempts to describe the direction of preference toward male or female sexual objects; (2) sexual interest, describing the intensity of attraction toward either object; and (3) sexual evaluation, describing the level of esteem placed on any sexual behaviour or interest.

We recognize that any such categories are arbitrary; those given above are described simply as alternatives for the reader. For the purposes of this chapter, however, three categories will be used : (1) self-reports of sexual experience or behaviour records; (2) self-reports of sexual arousal; (3) self-reports of sexual experience or arousal. Techniques used in each of these categories are most usually paper-and-pencil assessments in the form of a brief "test" or a behaviour record sheet to be filled in daily.

The most important assessment procedure used to collect self-report data on sexual behaviour is not a paper- and-pencil test ad runs across all three categories. It is the interview to assess sexual functioning, outlines for which have been suggested by many sex researchers. Masters and johnson outline specific questions to be asked during an interview and a specific sequence for asking the questions. They note that the tone of the interview, however, should be left to the clinical judgment of the therapist. The structured interview sets the occasion for more objective means of assessing sexual behaviour with the introduction of questions that can be asked repeatedly as therapy progresses. Since so many clinicians continue to rely on the interview to assess progress, developments in this area must be taken seriously. Birk, Huddleston, Miller, and Cohler and Bancroft also discuss the interview as a means of assessing sexual behaviour. In addition, numerous case history outlines have been constructed and are in common use in sex clinics around the country.

One of the best discussions of sex interviewing occurs in recent book by Caird and Wincze . Although the book is directed primarily toward sexual dysfunction rather than sexual deviation or deviation of gender role, the interview techniques described would be similar. Caird and Wincze discuss interviewing the female and interviewing the female in separate chapters and touch on such issues as the behaviour of the therapist in the interview, the type of language a therapist should use (i.e., clinical language or "street" language). and the effect of the sex of the interviewer on the patient. The necessity to be accepting and at ease with sexual material as well as the ability to use both clinical and street language greatly enhances the quality and quantity of data one may gather from these interviews, according to Caird and Wincze. Sample interviews provided in their book are useful to the beginning interviewer.

Self-report of sexual experiences and behaviour records: Podell and Perkins constructed a scale of 15 heterosexual activities ranging from "embrace" to "oral contact with female genitalia." Their hypothesis that subjects would not experience behaviours higher on the scale until they had first experience lower items was confirmed by a sample of 100 male college students. Similar scales were conducted by Brady and Levitt, Zuckerman, and Bentler. Bentler's scales, constructed for both males and females, were subjected to a sophisticated statistical analysis that demonstrated internal consistency. A cross-validation sample supported the generality of the scale. Essentially all these scales attempt to represent a normal progression of sexual experience. Treatment of those patients who are deficient in sexual behaviour should being about a chage in the score derived from such a scale. The data on self- report response modes are similar to those Geer and his associates are attempting to develop in the physiological response mode. These measures can be valuable or gathering information on change in sexual experience, but they are rather insensitive to the range and variety of sexual experience and are not entirely suited to repeated use over the course of treatment. However, LoPiccolo and Steger add an evaluative component to their questionnaire so that patients will rate the various behavioural items on a continuum of pleasantness or unpleasantness.

In our own research patients keep detailed behaviour records of several aspects of their sexual functioning. Simple form are constructed on which the patient can record all instances of sexual experience, all instances of masturbation and the fantasies accompanying masturbation, and all sexual fantasies occurring independently of sexual behaviour or masturbation. These records are constructed so that they are convenient to carry one's person and are coded to the patient's usual sexual experience. In most instances the patient must simply make a mark in the appropriate column. Since these records are individualized, the psychometric qualities of this type of record keeping cannot be determined. However, the purpose is not to compare the records with other patient's records but to examine changes over time in a given patient.

Self-Report measures of Sexual Arousal: Included in self-reports of sexual arousal are questionnaires that attempt to assess patterns of sexual arousal, often called sexual orientation or sexual interest. One of the best known methods of measuring patterns of sexual arousal is the sexual orientation method devised by Feldman. MacCulloch, Mellor, and Pinschoff. This scale was designed to measure changes in homosexual and heterosexual arousal patterns during treatment of males. The method has prompted a fair amount of research on its psychometric qualities . Feldman and MacCulloch stated that the scale was internally consistent an that test retest reliability was satisfactory. One difficulty with this scale was an early inclination by the authors to arbitrarily assign the label of "improved" or "cured" to a patient after a small amount of change on the scale. Although the scale does have end points in exclusive heterosexuality or exclusive homosexuality (within the limitation of self-report of arousal patterns) change within those boundaries is relative. Another difficulty is that the method is somewhat hard to score. Nevertheless, this instrument is used in our laboratories and is a helpful addition to out overall assessment program. Sambrooks and MacCulloch describe its use in a clinical setting in some detail. The Belfast group have modified the sexual orientation somewhat to include scale indicating anxiety as well as interest in different aspects of sexual behaviour. The revised versions have also been subjected to the usual psychometric procedures.

More recently, Hoon, Hoon, and Wincze have developed an inventory to measure female sexual arousal that is called the SAI. The inventory consists of 28 items describing erotic experiences which a respondent rates along a seven-point Likert-like scale or arousal, and it is as much an attitudinal scale as a method of reporting arousal. The advantage of this scale, according to its originators, is that it is easy to administer and score, has has good test/retest reliability, and may be used for single, married, and lesbian woman. Concurrent and discriminate validity have also been established. At present this seems to be the only scale applicable to single women.

Self-report of sexual attitudes: The LoPiccolo and Steger scale and the Hoon, Hoon, and Wincze inventory both qualify as attitudinal measures of sexual behaviour in the categorization adopted for this chapter, since they share an evaluative component. The Hoon, Hoon, and Wincze inventory is used exclusively with women, whereas the LoPiccolo and Steger is applicable only to heterosexual couples. Marks and Sartorius have published a sexual attitude scale based on the semantic differential technique. This sexual has been used primarily with sexual deviates and contains both sexual and nonsexual concepts that are rated on 13 bipolar scales,. Marks and Sartorius report that the sexual concepts are useful for assessing changes in the evaluation of deviant sexual attitudes, and they give examples of its use with transvestites and fetishists.

Other scales have been developed to evaluate anxiety associated with various sexual behaviours exclusively rather than as part of a larger scale. Although scales such as this do not assess sexual behavior directly, they may be useful in a comprehensive assessment. A good example is a scale constructed by Obler.

In our own laboratories a card sort method has been devised that, like the behaviour record used by Herman *et al.*, is highly individualized and therefore has not been subjected to psychometric evaluation. In the card sort method a series of sexual "scenes" is constructed. These scenes usually reflect the patient's experience, real or fantasized , with the sexual objects or situations in question. For example, in one experiment the patient was a 25-year-old, married pedophiliac. One scene in his card sort read, "You are alone in a room with a very sexy looking 10-year old girl with long blond hair." For the transsexual in the Barlow, Reynolds, and Agras article where propensity towards mistaken gender identity was the goal of assessment one scene card read, "I want to have female genitals." As many scenes as are relevant may be constructed and typed on three- by-five - inch cards. A similar set of scenes reflecting heterosexual arousal, masculine gender identity, or any other concept one wishes to assess can also be constructed. Everyday, or as often as desired, the patient takes the cards and sorts them into five envelopes marked to 4. He is instructed, "The numbers on these envelopes represent the amount of sexual arousal you experience" (in the case of assessment of patterns of sexual arousal) or "how much you desire this situation or set of circumstances at this time" (in the case of gender identity concepts). Zero equals none at all, one equals a little, two a fair amount, three much, and four very much. If he then put one card in the No. 4 envelope and one in No. 3, his score to that point would be 7, and so on. Caird and Wincze have adopted this procedure for individual assessment of sexual dysfunction. The obvious advantage of this procedure is its flexibility in that one can assess the strength of idiosyncratic attitudes concerning sexual concepts over time. Thus far this chapter has reviewed the sexual arousal behaviour in both contrived and natural situations in all three response modalities—the verbal, the motoric, and the physiological.

sexual conditioning the development of a positive mental attitude towards sexual activity as a normal human function, as opposed to the negative concept that anything sexual is wicked or nasty and may be tolerated only in certain situations, such as producing an offspring.

sexual cord a strand of cells in the embryo that give rise during foetal development to the follicles of the ovary and the seminiferous tubules of the testis.

sexual cosmetics cosmetics as a means of enhancing sexual attractiveness. Eye and face makeup are common in Western societies, but this form of ornamentation reached a peak in Eastern societies, particularly in ancient Egypt, China, and India. In particular, Tantric rites specify that a symbolic Third Eye be painted on the forehead to represent awakened consciousness; that body makeup consist of crushed marijuana, opium, and other intoxicating substances mixed with oils and pigments; and that the hands and feet of the woman be completely painted with designs.

sexual deprivation denial of an opportunity to obtain full sexual gratification as in prison, long sea voyages of males, and POW camps. One of the effects is deprivation homosexuality'; another is increase in emotional tension that cannot be adequately relieved by masturbation.

sexual desire an urgent need for sexual activity and gratification. According to Kinsey, this need reaches a peak among males during adolescence, and somewhat later among females. Though the urgency of the drive tends to decrease with age, it is usually present in some degree throughout life. Many couples, however, seek sex therapy or counselling when one member of the pair exhibits considerably less desire for sexual activity than the other. Many other couples consider themselves happily married even though they do not have a strong sexual desire and do not engage in frequent sexual activity.

sexual disorders any physical or psychological impairment of the ability to perform intercourse or produce offspring, because of such conditions as disease, injury, anatomical defect, internal conflict, or unconscious inhibition. Examples are impotence, frigidity, inhibited male or female orgasm, inhibited sexual excitement, dyspareunia, vaginismus, venereal diseases, cystitis, and cancer of the cervix or prostate.

sexual display the endless ways of exhibiting sexual features to enhance sexual attractiveness. In our culture, women rely largely on cosmetics, hair fashions, deep necklines, slit skirts or miniskirts, designer jeans, long boots, and revealing bikinis. Many men rely on body-hugging trousers, shirts, and extremely small bathing suits. In some super masculine groups, men artificially enlarge their muscles by 'Pumping iron' or wear leather clothing and studded belts to arouse sexual fantasies. Societies in 'underdeveloped, countries have their own means of sexual display such as tattooing, scarification, large penis sheaths, body piercing, and depilation.

sexual dreams dream sequences involving sexual activities, attractive members of the opposite sex, images of sexual features, and sexual symbols. Sexual dreams are frequently a key to the individual's sexual desires, concerns, and frustrations. Such dreams may be accompanied by erection and ejaculation in boys and men, and by vaginal lubrication and orgasm in women. The term sexual dreams is usually distinguished from SEX DREAMS.

sexual dwarf a misleading term for a dwarf who is an adult with normally developed adult genitalia.

sexual dysfunction a sexual malfunction that interferes with adequate sexual performance and gratification, because of psychological physiological factors or both. Masters and Johnson maintain that some form of sexual inadequacy or dysfunctioning is found in at least 50 percent of American marriages. Examples are dysparcunia, impotence, premature ejaculation, retarded ejaculation, vaginismus, retrograde ejaculation, ejaculatory incompetence, inhibited sexual desire, inhibited sexual excitement, inhibited female orgasm, and inhibited male orgasm.

sexual ecstasy the peak of pleasure, excitement, and euphoria experienced at the moment of orgasm, or climax.

sexual excitement the first phase of the sexual response cycle, in which sexual stimuli of various kinds-fondling, kissing, tonguing, looking, and sometimes sucking-produce a state of tension and arousal. During this state, vaginal lubrication, swelling of the labia, and erection of the nipples and clitoris occur in the female, and erection of the penis and contraction of the scrotum take place in the male, while increased blood flow and heart rate occur in both. Sexual excitement can also be produced by fantasies, masturbation, sex dreams, dancing, and the rhythmical movements of a vehicle.

sexual exploitation taking advantage of another person or persons for sexual purposes, either as a source of financial gain or for personal gratification. Major forms of sexual exploitation are enticing boys and girls into heterosexual or homosexual prostitution, using them as subjects for pornographic films and magazines, and forcing them into pederasty and sodomy.

sexual failure in the male, failure to achieve or maintain erection, premature ejaculation, or failure to ejaculate; in the female, failure to be aroused, painful intercourse, or failure to reach orgasm; in both, failure to derive pleasure from sexual activity.

sexual fantasies erotic images of either standard lovemaking or, in about 25 percent of instances, such variations as homosexual encounters, group sex, or sadomasochism. Recent studies indicate that most people have seven or eight such fantasies every day, and that replacement of the established partner, forced sexual encounters, and observation of the sexual activities of others are three of the most common. They are not necessarily a key to one's basic sexual orientation, but they may reveal a need for psychotherapy, as in cases where there are problems of intimacy, or an obsession with rape and sadistic images.

sexual favours an obsolescent term for sexual 'privileges,' including intercourse and other activities, granted by women, usually freely but sometimes for remuneration. Men, too, may grant sexual favours to women or other men.

sexual fears various fears that affect sexual performance and gratification, including fear of inadequacy; fear of not arousing or satisfying one's partner, fear of pregnancy, fear of injury, fear of discovery, fear of contracting a venereal disease, and, in psychoanalytical theory, an unconscious castration fear among men.

sexual fetish a fetish that involves part of the body associated with reproduction, such as the breasts or genitals.

sexual flush suffusion of skin areas with blood during sexual excitement particularly in women. Flushing begins with a rashlike discoloration of the lower chest, and spreads to the breasts and the rest of the chest and neck, reaching a peak in the late plateau phase just before orgasm, rapidly subsiding during the resolution phase of the sexual response cycle.

sexual frustration thwarting of the sexual impulse in greater or lesser degree, by such internal forces as parental admonitions, the demands of religion, feelings of insecurity or anxiety, and such external circumstances as confinement to prison, rigid social rules, or lack of opportunity to meet members of the opposite sex or a partner with a lower sex drive.

sexual fulfilment the sense of completion and gratification that follows a successful sexual encounter. Fulfilment is experienced in the orgasmic and resolution phases of the sexual response cycle.

sexual functioning the performance of sexual intercourse, or the ability to perform intercourse.

sexual gratification satisfaction of the sex urge, usually implying orgasm. The term is a broad one covering any form of intercourse and any other means of achieving sexual excitement and release, such as flagellation, masturbation, or sadistic activities.

sexual gymnastics a term applied to extreme, highly athletic forms of sexual activity, such as copulation on or in a chariot, as illustrated in early Egyptian, Hindu, and Japanese manuscripts.

sexual harassment unwanted sexual attentions usually from men towards women.

sexual history a compilation of detailed information on a patient's sexual behaviour and experiences throughout his or her past and present life. A sexual history is usually an integral part of a psychological case history assembled for purposes of diagnosis and prognosis in psychiatry or clinical psychology, because many cases of mental disorder involve disturbed sexual relationships.

sexual humour riddles, songs, tall tales, limericks, jokes, and other comic material that involve a reference to sexual anatomy or sexual activity. Psychologically, laughter at such humour is believed to arise not only from the display of wit, but from an urge to defy social conventions or a need to release inner repressions, or what Freud has called 'letting the cat out of the bag'.

sexual identity a person's biologically determined sex orientation; the internal sense of maleness or femaleness. In cases of ambiguous genitalia, as in hermaphroditism, the individual may be confused about his or her sexual identity.

sexual inadequacy inability to achieve a satisfactory level of sexual satisfaction, and to help ones partner to achieve a similar level. Masters and Johnson have estimated that at least 50 percent of marriages are afflicted with some form of sexual inadequacy or dysfunctioning, such as lack of desire, inability to reach or enjoy orgasm, impotence, or frigidity. Other specialists have reported that as many as 75 percent of their patients have sexual problems severe enough to require professional help.

sexual incompatibility inability of sexual partners to adjust to each other's needs, stemming from such factors as differences in sexual desire or timing, impotence or frigidity, physical disability, anatomical incongruity, inhibitions or other emotional 'hangups' on the part of one or both partners. Sexual incompatibility is grounds for divorce in some countries.

sexual infantilism the tendency to avoid forms of

sexual expression characteristic of adults, especially intercourse, and to limit oneself to activities that were appropriate during the years of childhood, such as stroking, biting, and kissing. Many psychosexual disorders, including fetishism and voyeurism, are considered basically infantile.

sexual inhibition an unconscious, involuntary suppression of the sexual impulse, especially the inability to feel sexual desire, to perform adequately, or to experience orgasm. The condition results from such factors as fear of failure or injury, or negative feelings implanted by the parents.

sexual instincts a psychoanalytical term for all erotic drives, anal, oral, and genital. Freud held that these instincts not only afford pleasure and lead to preservation of the species, but may also be 'sublimated' into creative activities such as artistic and scientific pursuits. Sexual instincts is also a biological term for all unlearned behaviour involved in sexual activities and reproduction, such as nest building, courtship behaviour, and copulation in animals.

sexual intercourse the commonly expression for the more technical term coitus.

sexuality the capacity to behave sexually, that is, to respond to erotic stimuli and to obtain pleasure from sexual activities such as foreplay, intercourse, and masturbation. Sexuality involves not only the genital organs but all the erogenous zones of the body, as well as all wishes, desires, and fantasies associated with sex.

sexualization the process of endowing various parts of the body and various activities with sexual energy, which Freud termed the libido.

Psychoanalysts would also include all types of behaviour into which sexual energy is 'sublimated,' such as creative art and scientific research.

sexualization of society the preoccupation with sex in various cultures; the pervasive effects of sexual interests, customs, and behaviour on a given culture, as exemplified by the influence of sex-oriented films and magazines in Western society and the influence of sexual mysticism in Eastern societies.

sexual liberation a trend towards (a) greater freedom of sexual expression, which had hitherto been hampered by the repressive Morality of the Victorian era, and (b) greater freedom in sexual research, which had hitherto been hampered by prejudice, ignorance, and reliance on folklore and superstition. Among the great liberators on both counts are Havelock Ellis, Hirschfeld, Krafft-Ebing, Freud, Margaret Sanger, Marie Stopes, Kinsey, and Masters and Johnson.

sexual life-style the, particular pattern of sexual expression developed by each individual on the basis of his or her experience with sexual relationships, individual sexual needs and desires, and male or female sex role. Sexual life-styles vary all the way from the prudishness of the Puritan to the licentiousness of the libertine.

sexually mature female from the anatomical point of view, a woman whose primary sex organs and secondary sex characteristics are fully developed.

sexually mature male from the anatomical point of view, a man whose primary sex organs and secondary sex characteristics are fully developed.

sexually transmitted disease (STD) any disease that may be acquired by sexual contact with another person, including AIDS; balanitis gangraenosa; candidiasis; chancroid, chlamydia; crab louse; cytomegalovirus, genital herpes, genital warts; gonorrhoea; granuloma inguinale group B streptococcal infection; hepatitis B herpes simplex 1; herpes simplex 2; lymphogranuloma venereum ; molluscum contagiosum; nongonococcal urethritis, Reiter's disease; scabies; syphilis, trichomoniasis; and yaws.

The term venereal disease is more popular but less precise than sexually transmitted disease.

sexual maladjustment any condition of failure to achieve normal sexual relations with another person, as manifested in impotence, frigidity, vaginismus, or other sexual problems.

sexual marketplace a general term for the group of individual enterprises that make a business of sex, including houses of prostitution, massage parlours, 'adult' book shops, shops that specialize in sex aids, pimping, pornographic films, and magazines that specialize in sexually explicit articles and photographs.

sexual masochism the term used by the American Psychiatric Association for a psychosexual disorder in which sexual arousal is repeatedly or exclusively sought through being beaten, flogged, bound, verbally abused, or otherwise maltreated, or through voluntary participation in an activity that involves being subjected to physical harm or threat to life.

sexual maturation the development of the reproductive system to the point where intercourse and reproduction are possible. Also called sexual maturity.

sexual mechanisms the physical structures and functions involved in sexual activity, including the internal and external sex organs, reflexes, muscles that control coital postures and movements, and the sex hormones involved in erection, ejaculation, vaginal secretions, and orgasm.

sexual melanchollа a mentally depressed state, ohm part of a bipolar disorder, in which a male is convinced that he is impotent.

sexual myths misconceptions and fallacies arising out of hearsay, superstition, bigotry, or faulty sexual education. Examples are the beliefs that alcohol is a sexual stimulant that women who have multiple orgasms tend to be oversexed; that hormonal imbalance is the major cause of homosexuality; that a seventh month baby has a better chance for survival than an eight-month baby; that sexually frigid women are less likely to conceive than responsive women; that a prostatectomy reduces sexual capability; or that masturbation produces debility and mental disorder.

sexual need an internal condition of tension generated by an unsatisfied desire for sexual gratification. The basis for this need is three fold: biological, psychological, and social. Even though sexual need has a physical basis and is sometimes called metaphorically sexual 'hunger,' and although at times'people as well as animals may prefer copulation to eating, sexual activity is not necessary to sustain life except in a broad sense of species Preservation. Moreover, the need is conditioned by such factors as opportunity, the attractiveness and willingness of the partner, the social situation, and the desire for release of tension created by work or worry.

sexual negativism a term applied by Magnus Hirschfeld to a lack of interest in sex that might stem from a deficit of sexual hormones.

sexual neuroses neurotic trends and symptoms that have a sexual basis. Among these are inordinate sexual desire sexual anxiety, excessive sexual submissiveness or timidity, extreme prudishness stemming from feelings of guilt instilled in childhood, compulsive sex activity as a compensation for feelings of inferiority, extreme preoccupation with sexual fantasies, phobias related to sex, and sexual dysfunctions resulting from deep-seated emotional conflicts and tensions.

sexual nightmare a vivid dream depicting an acutely disturbing anxiety-provoking sexual encounter. Typically, the dreamer is caught in a threatening situation such as being attacked by a rapist, experiences agonizing dread, makes futile attempts to escape, and awakens in a cold sweat.

sexual normality sexual behaviour that is considered acceptable within a particular culture or population,

sexual norms the accepted standards of sexual attitudes and behaviour. These standards vary widely from society to society and from time to time. In one society sex may be regarded as d marital duty (especially by the wife); in another, sexual gratification is considered a right for the woman as well as the man. In one social group, 'recreational sex' (including swinging) is the norm;

in another, any departure from traditional behaviour (for example, from the missionary position) is considered taboo.

sexual novelty sexual activity with new partners, or in untried ways, usually as a means of satisfying curiosity or escaping from boredom or monotony. The search for novelty is most likely to occur when the established partner is unimaginative, inhibited, or uninterested in experimentation.

sexual oralism a type of sexual activity in which partners obtain pleasure by applying the mouth, lips, or tongue to the sex organs of the other individual. Studies indicate an association between a desire for sexual oralism and a sensitivity for certain aromas associated with the genitalia. The activity is not considered deviant if it is not performed to the exclusion of other forms of sexual pleasure.

sexual orientation an established pattern of sexual interest and in most cases sexual activity directed towards members of the other sex (heterosexuality), the same sex (homosexuality), or both sexes (bisexuality). The orientation Pattern usually becomes fixed during the first few years of life.

sexual-orientation disturbance an older psychiatric category comprising individuals whose sexual interests are directed towards persons of the same sex, and who are emotionally disturbed by this orientation. In the current classification of mental disorders by the American Psychiatric Association, this category has been replaced by the term egodystonic homosexuality.

sexual outlet any form of behaviour that results in the release of sexual tension, especially through the achievement of orgasm. Examples are 'heavy' petting, masturbation, nocturnal emissions, and all forms of intercourse including fellatio, curmilingus, and anal coitus.

sexual pathology sexual aberrations and disorders, such as those described in KrafftEbing's monumental work, *Psychopathia Sexualis.* Major examples are sadism, masochism, syphilis and other venereal diseases, impotence, frigidity, genital mutilation, coprophilia, necrophilia, satyriasis, and nymphomania.

sexual permissiveness the view that sexual activity should be as free as possible from restrictions or regulations, based on the conviction that sexual expression and experimentation are natural and good. The permissive attitude countenances such practices as orogenital contact and recreational sex, among adults, and usually favours legalization of abortion and recognition of homosexual relationships among consenting adults. It rarely if ever favours elimination of controls on such practices as paedophilia; rape, extreme sadomasochism, and incest, nor does it favour sexual irresponsibility and exploitation.

sexual perversion a culturally unacceptable deviation from prevailing norms of sexual behaviour.

sexual phobias intense, morbid fears stemming from sexual inhibitions, neuroses, or traumatic experiences. They include fear of sex after rape, or injury (traumatophobia), of women (gynaephobia), of homosexuals, (homophobia), or bearing a monster (teratophobia), of being touched (haptephobia), of childbirth (maieusiophobia), of female genitals (eurotophobia), of girls (parthenophobia), of men (androphobia), of marriage (gamophobia), of naked bodies (gymnophobia), of pleasure (hedonophobia), of pointed objects including penises and penis symbols (aichmophobia), of semen (spermatophobia), of sex generally (genophobia), of sexual intercourse (coitophobia), of snakes (ophidiophobia), of syphilis (syphilophobia), and of venereal disease generally (cypriphobia).

sexual pleasure the sense of pleasure experienced through sexual stimulation or gratification, as in necking and petting, foreplay, masturbation, any type of intercourse, viewing sexual films and photographs, watching other people engaged in sexual activity, reading erotic books and articles, using devices designed to enhance sexual response, and engaging in unusual Practices that stimulate sexual response, such as bondage and flagellation.

sexual precocity premature development of primary and secondary sex characteristics. In boys, sexual precocity may stem from early development of centres in the hypothalamus, or from dysfunctions of the adrenal cortex or the interstitial cells of the testes. In girls, neoplasms in or on the ovaries may affect hormonal output and produce rapid and premature enlargement of the breasts. Premature development of the genitalia, and early growth of pubic hair.

sexual preference Preference for sexual activity with males, females, or both, or for specific forms of sexual gratification such as oral sex, anal sex, rear entry, woman-above, man-above, mutual masturbation, as well as for particular forms of sexual stimulation such as biting, whipping, and bondage.

sexual preoccupation a strong, sometimes obsessive,

interest in or concern about sex. An obvious example is the large role played by sex in Western clothing styles, novels, art, films, and the mass media. But any examination of Eastern cultures, such as Hindu and Polynesian societies, indicates an equal or even greater preoccupation with sex. Moreover, sexual preoccupation is also exemplified by negative attitudes, such as those expressed in Christianity, in Victorian society, in cultures like Inis Beag, and among prudes and other sexual zealots.

sexual primordial reaction a term introduced by Wilhelm Stekel to describe the normal behaviour of appraising any other person in terms of 'sexual worth.' Stekel related the human behaviour to that observed in lower animals, such as dogs sniffing each other a, their first meeting. Stekel commented, Consciously or unconsciously we disrobe every stranger with whom we become acquainted and form an image of the stranger's genitalia.'

sexual problems a wide range of difficulties, dysfunctions, and psychosocial disorders associated with sexual adjustment. Typical male problems include impotence, feelings of inadequacy, premature ejaculation, priapism, inhibited sexual desire, inhibited orgasm, incest, sexual sadism, child molestation, fetishism, voyeurism, bestiality, exhibitionism, transvestism, necrophilia, rape, confusion over sexual orientation or gender identity, and satyriasis. Typical female problems include frigidity, inhibited orgasm, dyspareunia, vagmismus, nymphomania, confusion over sexual orientation or gender identity, inhibited sexual desire, exhibitionism, transvestism, child molestation, sexual masochism, and fetishism.

sexual proceptivity the female's tendency to be attracted to males and to act as a sexual stimulus for males Studies show that secretion of the hormone oestrogen produces proceptive behaviour ranging from merely approaching, investigating, and staying near the male, to explicit invitations or solicitations of copulation. This has been shown to occur in animals such as dogs, rodents, and monkeys, and may occur in women as well.

sexual prodigies a term sometimes applied to individuals who display or are reputed to display a high level of sexual activity. Among the most celebrated are the Roman Empress Valeria Messalina and Emperor Nero in the Ist century, and Catherine II of Russia and the Venetian Casanova in the 18th century, Also Goethe, greatest of German writers, almost certainly made many thousands of sexual conquests; and in our time, Georges Simenon asserts he made love to at least 10,000 women (or about three women per week on average in six decades of sexual pursuit-besides writing over 500 novels. However, frequent sexual activity is also found among ordinary people (who generally just don't talk about it). Kinsey's studies reveal that 7 percent of (white American) males averaged seven orgasms per week, and one man averaged 33 per week over 30 years. Kinsey also found that generally women were as active as males.

sexual prowess unusual skill and endurance in the physical art of lovemaking, with particular emphasis on frequency of intercourse. Display of sexual prowess is the major motive among satyriasists and nymphomaniacs, as well as in certain primitive societies, such as the Chaga of

Tanzania, where it is not unusual for men to have intercourse as often as 10 times a night.

sexual psychopath an individual with an antisocial personality whose characteristic offences take the form of repeated sexual aggression such as rape, child molestation, or sexual mutilation, as well as nonviolent activities such as exhibitionism, bestiality, and incest.

sexual receptivity the readiness of females to be 'receptive to the sexual advances of males. In female animals, receptivity is highest during the oestrus; in human females, it tends to be highest just before and just after menstruation, although responsiveness is not wholly determined by physiological mechanisms. Among the other factors involved are the attractiveness of the male and his skill as a sexual partner, as well as the setting in which his advances are made.

sexual reflex the erection of the genitalia and orgasm or ejaculation as a result of physical or psychic erotic stimulation, or both.

sexual reflexes any of a number of spontaneous physical responses to a stimulus that may have an erotic effect. Included are the abdominal reflex, produced by stroking the skin overlying the abdominal wall; the bulbospongiosus reflex, produced by tapping the top of the penis; the cremasteric reflex, caused by stimulating the skin on the inside of the male thigh; and Geigel's reflex, in which stroking the skin of the female thigh causes a response similar to the cremasteric reflex in the male.

sexual regression an event in embryonic life that follows the first sign that the indifferent sex organs will become either male or female genitalia. Until the time that sexuality is determined, the embryo exhibits sex ducts that may become either male or female organs. During the seventh week of gestation, one set of sex ducts will advance beyond the indifferent state, and the complementary set of ducts, either male or female, will undergo regression.

sexual rehabilitation restoration of the ability to function sexually by treating a sexual dysfunction such as impotence, vaginismus, or rape-trauma syndrome. The term applies also to measures taken to enable a disabled person, such as a quadriplegic, to function sexually as well as possible.

sexual rejuvenation the restoration of youthful sexual vigour among the aging. An untold number of substances, exercises, and treatments have been tried and found wanting. Among them are downright frauds such as radioactive water, x-ray lamps, and various pills and lotions, as well as substances that might, just might, have aphrodisiac effects, as palmetto seeds, soma-plant extract and Spanish fly, Various pseudomedical treatments are also prevalent including gland transplants of goat and monkey testes; unilateral vasectomy: the cellular therapy of Paul Niehans, a Swiss physician; and a procaine containing drug developed by Professor Anna Asian of Rumania, which may have a greater tranquillizing than rejuvenating effect.

sexual repression in psychoanalysis, a defence mechanism in which unacceptable sexual impulses are banned from consciousness because they produce anxiety; also, deliberate attempts to curb sexual activity and sexual interest as in extremely Puritanical or other sexually inhibited societies.

sexual response reaction to sexual stimulation such as fondling or kissing. Initial responses of females include vaginal lubrication and erection of the nipples. In males, the most obvious response is erection of the penis. Responsiveness is determined by such factors as sexual desire and readiness, environmental circumstances, the skill of the partner, and the use of stimulants.

sexual-response cycle the generalized Pattern of sexual response as reported by Masters and Johnson, which is applicable not only to heterosexual intercourse, but to homo-sexual and masturbatory activities as well. The four stages of this cycle are excitement, plateau, orgasm, and resolution.

sexual response time the amount of time required for the average man or woman to reach orgasm. Some studies indicate that a man needs between 2 and 4 minutes to reach SEXUAL REVOLUTION orgasm while, despite the general belief that a woman requires more time, some women have been found to reach orgasm in as little as 15 to 30 seconds while the average is less than 4 minutes.

Sexual revolution the widespread shift in sexual attitudes and behaviour in the direction of greater permissiveness, more liberal attitudes towards premarital sex, assertion of women's sexual rights and needs, revolt against the double standard, frank and open sex education, more varied sexual relations and sexual activity at earlier ages than at the start of this century. These changes may be characterized as a revolution when compared with the Victorian era, but studies show that the change is often more in attitudes than in actions, and that extremes like group sex and swinging have not become standard sexual behaviour.

sexual rights as used in cross-cultural studies, a term that usually refers to the exercise of sexual privileges with women other than a man's wife-for example, the right to intercourse with the wife's sister, the right a, brothers to sexual access to each other's wives, or the right of the father of a newly married man to initial intercourse with his son's wife.

sexual script an individual's unique pattern of attitudes and expectations concerning sexual behaviour responses, roles, feelings, and relationships. The script' reflects not only individual experiences, but the influence of the persons family, culture, and subculture

sexual selection the Darwinian concept that the choice of a mate is based on attractive features such as the coloration or song d birds. This process, which-has its counterpart in human beings, tends to favour reproduction of individuals with similar attractive traits.

Sexual senescence the gradual decline in sexual functions during the later years of life especially in women after menopause, whet the reproductive cycle is slowly extinguished and after the climacteric among men whet potency and fertility slowly diminish. However, sexual interest may continue indefinitely.

sexual sorcery attempts of witch doctors and shamans to enlist supernatural powers by the use of spells, incantations, black magic, and drugs, for such purposes as enforcement of sexual taboos, sexual rejuvenation, and cure of sexual ills such as impotence.

sexual standards norms of sexual behaviour as set by a particular society or subculture, or by particular influences such as parental teachings, moral or religious beliefs and dicta, civil laws, superstitions, the mass media. It is often said that almost every form of sexual behaviour has been condemned or condoned in some place at some time. Kinsey has pointed out that most people desire many outlets for their sexuality, that virtually everyone behaves sexually in some manner condemned by society or probably by laws as well.

sexual stimulation any form of stimulation that produces sexual excitement: tactile, visual, psychological, orogenital contact, anal penetration, and various other forms of heterosexual and homosexual intercourse.

sexual synergism the collaboration of different, and sometimes contradictory, stimuli to produce sexual excitement. Freud maintained that these stimuli may include unpleasant as well as pleasant stimuli (fright, horror, or pain), or even a combination of love and hate, provided these do not exceed a certain limit.

sexual taboo a sexual act, word, or symbol that is prohibited in a particular society on religious or social grounds. Most common, though not universal, are incest taboos, followed by prohibitions against semi intercourse during menstruation, pregnancy, and nursing. In various parts of Africa, intercourse is prohibited during daylight hours, before going to war, during a thunderstorm, and for up to a year after birth of a child. Elsewhere there are taboos against sex between grandparents (a Taiwan Society), on birthdays of the gods (traditional Chinese), after planting narcotic plants (Ivaro Indians), against intercourse out of doors (among the Yucatec and Mayan Indians) and indoors (in Papua New Guinea), as well as during certain phases of the moon (Hindu societies). In West ern society, adultery, anal intercourse, sex with animals, and the use of certain gestures and certain slang words for sex organs and activities are frequently considered taboo.

sexual techniques activities that enhance or inhibit sexual arousal in one's partner. Sex educators generally agree that there has recently been an overemphasis on 'technique' in the sense of specific behaviour that is bound to produce a maximum response Instead, they say that the emphasis should be on experimenting with various approaches, discovering what both partners like, and communicating special desires to each other. Any number of activities can be either positive or negative in their effect on a particular relationship deep or light kissing, lightly biting different parts of the partner's body, deep or shallow penetration, cuddling and fondling, making love silently or expressing one's feelings openly, or emphasizing or deemphasizing simultaneous orgasm. In any case there are no set rules and recommendations, except to be imaginative spontaneous, and to focus on one's partner's pleasure as well as one's own.

sexual tension a condition of restlessness and strain resulting from an acute desire or need for sexual gratification and release, usually relieved by experiencing orgasm.

sexual trauma an emotionally disturbing sexual experience such as rape, sexual child abuse, incest, or forced anal intercourse. Experiences of this kind are psychologically injurious and may result in marked feelings of anxiety, sexual phobias, inhibited sexual desire, or inability to reach orgasm.

sexual underactivity the Level of sexual activity that is at the lower end of the frequency.

sexual vandalism a compulsion to destroy sexual features depicted in statues, painting, or other art forms.

sexual variance sexual behaviour that varies from what is considered conventional or usual. It may be manifested in the choice of a sex partner or object, in the degree and strength of the sexual drive, and in the method of functioning and quality of sexual striving.

sexy erotically provocative, suggestive stimulating, as applied to a person, film, novel, photograph, or play. It can also mean aroused, horny or randy.

shock up a colloquial term meaning to live like husband and wife without being legally married.

shaft a slang term meaning to copulate with a woman.

shag a slang term meaning to copulate. By extension shagged out means extremely tired.

shagbag a derogatory slang term for a woman of loose sexual morals, particularly one whose activities in this area over the years have left their mark on her appearance.

shagger's back a humorous Australian slang term for bad backache.

Shakespearean terms with sexual meanings an extraordinary number of terms—over 1,500—with direct or implied sexual meanings that occur in the works of the greatest author of the English language. Most of these terms were common 400 years ago, but many were coined by Shakespeare. His sexually most risque works include *Much Ado about Nothing, The Merry Wives of Windsor, Hamlet, Measure for Measure, Othello, and Henry the Fifth,* and in *Romeo and Juliet* there is a passage of 23 lines that includes no fewer than 12 different sexual terms, mainly for male and female genitalia and for intercourse. Many of Shakespeare's sex-related terms and puns are still in active use today.

shaman a 'medicine man,' priest or 'witch doctor' who uses sorcery' to cure mental or physical illness. In many Native American and Asian societies, shamans enforce sexual taboos such as intercourse in a cornfield, or abstention from intercourse for a year after taking a scalp. They themselves frequently abstain from sexual activity, Particularly when they are in training, and in the Siberian cultures many shamans are transvestites.

shame feelings of humiliation associated with exposure of one's faults and shortcomings; also, acute embarrassment experienced by some individuals over exposure of their genitals, or self-consciousness about menstruation or skin disorders during Puberty. Psychoanalysts claim that feelings of shame may be a defence against exhibitionist impulses.

shame-eversion therapy a form of behaviour therapy in which an undesirable activity, usually sexual in nature, is enacted before a neutral audience as a means of creating a sense of shame in the patient. The final objective is to encourage the patient to avoid such behaviour because of the shameful feelings it produces.

sheepshagger a British slang term for someone who sodomizes a sheep, particularly in the absence of any other sexual outlet. It came into vogue during the Falklands War as a derogatory term for the islanders, among˘ whose scattered population sheep-farming i a major occupation.

shoot-smell a slang term referring to a private eye's tailing someone to intimate situations to obtain evidence.

she-male a recent synonym for a butch especially in prison slang.

shirtlifter a derogatory term of Australia origin for a male homosexual.

shoo fetishism an obsession with shoes a sexual objects or symbols, as in retifism.

shoot a colloquial term meaning to ejaculate.

short-eyes an American prison-slang term for a child molester.

short hairs a colloquial term for pubic hairs When used in the phrase of 'having somebody by the short hairs,' the connotation is that one has another person under one's control or power.

shotgun perineum medical jargon for a congenital abnormality in some women in which the anus and vagina appear side by side.

shotgun wedding a slang term for a marriage necessitated by a pregnancy; a forced wedding.

show, the the plug of mucus in the neck of the womb of a pregnant woman which, when dislodged, can indicate the onset of labour.

shower cap an American slang term for condom.

showering in a raincoat an American slang term meaning intercourse with a condom.

shrimping an American slang term for sucking the Partner's toes for one's own and/or the Partner's sexual turn-on.

shut-eyes an American prison-slang term for a sex offender generally.

sibling one of two or more children who have a common parent. Siblings may be brothers, sisters, or both.

sibling rivalry competition among siblings for the attention, affection, or approval of one or both parents, or for recognition at school, or on the playing field.

side girl a married man's girlfriend. The term is popular throughout the English-speaking Caribbean but also in parts of the southeastern United States, especially in black English.

silent board an older term for a woman's pubic hair.

silent rape reaction a psychiatric syndrome that evolves from a rape that has not been reported to anyone. The symptoms are similar to those of the rape-trauma syndrome but often expressed as psychosomatic complaints, anxiety, or depression. Researchers believe that many women do not report rapes and as a result suffer from the symptoms of silent rape reaction.

Simmond's disease a chronic progressive hormonal disorder marked by signs and symptoms that include decreased sexual function and atrophy of the genitalia. The disease, which may affect both men and women, results in a loss of pubic and axillary hair, loss of facial hair in men, weight, loss, emaciation, hypoglycaemia, and signs of premature aging. The symptoms reflect failure of the anterior lobe of the Pituitary gland.

Sim's position a posture in which a patient lies on the left side with the right knee and thigh drawn upwards towards the chest. It is one of several Positions used for a medical examination of the male prostate gland.

simulsex a colloquial term for bisexuality.

simultaneous fertilization the fertilization of more than one ovum at approximately the same time by the spermatozoa of one or more males. The simultaneous fertilization will result in dizygotic twins, or in some instances triplets or quadruplets, depending upon the number of ova released at the same time. The tendency to release more than one ovum at the same time is an inherited trait of some women, but may also result from fertility drugs.

simultaneous orgasm an alternative term for mutual orgasm.

singles bar a bar that caters to unmarried men and women who are seeking entertainment, companionship, and, in many instances, sexual contacts.

sinning fear an intense, sometimes morbid fear of committing or having committed an unpardonable sin. In its pathological form, this phobia may be a symptom of mental illness. However, it may also be instilled by parents or others as a means of controlling sexual impulses, particularly the urge to masturbate. In psychiatry, sinning fear of the pathological sort has several names: peccatophobia, hamartophobia, and enosiophobia.

sister a male homosexual slang term for a fellow homosexual.

sister of the night a colloquial term for prostitute.

sit on the fence a colloquial term meaning to be bisexual.

situational homosexuality male or female homosexuality undertaken in an environment in which the opposite sex is inaccessible for a more or less extended period, such as in a boarding school, in a prison, aboard ship, or at a military outpost. Homosexuality of this kind may only be temporary, and heterosexual contacts may be resumed soon after release from the situation. Similarly used terms are accidental homosexuality, faute de mieux, and occasional inversion.

situational orgasmic dysfunction a term applied by Masters and Johnson to nonorgasmic women who have managed to reach orgasm at least once in their lives, whether by masturbation, coitus, or some other form of stimulation, but no longer do so.

69 a colloquial term for mutual oral sex: The partners assume a head-to-feet position and perform fellatio and cunnilingus simultaneously. The technique may be a prelude to intercourse, or may itself be a means of achieving orgasm.

66 a slang term for anal intercourse. Also written sixty-six. A synonymous term is '99'.

size queen a slang term used by male homosexuals to refer to a partner with large genitalia.

Skene's glands paraurethral glands located on either side of the urethral meatus of the female. They are believed to be vestiges of tissues that would have developed into the Prostate gland if the individual had differentiated into a male instead of a female. Skene's glands are often the site of inflammation if the person acquires gonorrhoea.

skin brassiere medical jargon for the Skin tissues of the breast that hold the breast in an appropriate position with aesthetic forward projection.

skin colour the colour of the skin as a component of sexual attractiveness. In the white 'race,' light-coloured skin is not universally prized, though alabaster sculpture may give that impression. In Victorian times, Western ladies carried parasols to avoid a suntan, but today a suntanned face and body are considered highly sexy, Attitudes vary greatly: Some Polynesians attempt to bleach their skin, but Trobrianders find both albinos and very dark people equally distasteful. Among dark-skinned people, many societies, countries, or individuals value the darkest shades as especially beautiful.

skin decoration in sexology, the decoration of the skin for sexual attractiveness. The almost universal use of makeup-heavy or light-in both Eastern and Western societies attests to the fact that skin decoration has sexual overtones, particularly among women. In non-Western societies, such as Zaire and Samoa, extensive tattoos, elaborate scars, and painted designs on the bodies of both men and women are considered highly erotic.

skin-dive a slang term meaning to perform curmilingus.

skin eroticism sexual excitement derived from caressing, rubbing, or licking the skin, especially during foreplay. Also, exposure of large areas of the skin can be stimulating in itself. It is no accident that pornographic films are called 'skin flicks.' The skin is regarded as a secondary sex organ, and Freud saw it as the erotogenic zone par excellence.

skin flick a colloquial term for a pornographic film; also, for a sexually explicit film that is not entirely pornographic.

skirt a slang term for women in general, considered as objects of sexual pursuit. It is used in such contexts as a piece of skirt and a skirt-chaser.

Skoptsy an ascetic religious sect dating from the 18th century and composed of dissenters from the Russian Orthodox Church. The name itself is derived from the Russian *skopets*, meaning eunuch, which aptly befits the cult's ritual of castration in which the scrotum and testicles are first removed, and afterwards the penis itself. This practice is based on their interpretation of a passage in the Book of Matthew: 'And there be eunuchs, which have made themselves eunuchs for the kingdom of heaven's sake. Some Skoptsy women participate in the ritual by having their ovaries and even their breast excised.

slap and tickle British rolloquial term for petting.

slash a British slang term for urination usually in the phrase 'have a slash.'

slaughterhouse an older slang term for brothel, especially a mass brothel.

sleep around to be promiscuous in one's sex life; have sex with many partners.

sleeping together a euphemism for nonmarital sex.

Some studies show, however, that significant percentage of young males am females may live together for several month before having intercourse.

sloop with a euphemism meaning to have intercourse with (someone). This euphemism has been in use for a thousand years.

slim a slang term for the external female genitals. Slim a name used for AIDS in East Africa, where the disease is rife. It is derived, with macabre irony, from the emaciation the disease causes.

slit a slang term for the external female genitals.

sloughing a condition in which immature male germ cells are released into the tubules leading to the epididymis. The immature cells are unable to progress normally and eventually clog the tubules. Because only a reduced number of mature spermatozoa are actually produced and released from the testes, the patient is usually diagnosed as lacking normal fertility because of oligospermia.

slut a dirty or immoral woman; also, a prostitute.

S/M abbreviation for sadomasochistic, that is, sadism with masochism.

smallest baby the smallest infant reported to have survived after birth. According to the Guinness Book of Records the tiniest viable infant weighed 10 ounces, delivered without the help of a doctor in England in 1938.

small-penis complex an emotional concern by some men that they possess a penis that is abnormally small, a concern based in part on the individual's visual perspective when looking downwards towards a flaccid penis, a viewpoint that distorts the true size. The complex may also be supported by the emphasis in literature and other art forms as well as folklore and pornographic material on male genitalia that are unusually large.

smegma a fatty or oily substance secreted by sebaceous glands of the prepuce and the neck and glands of the penis of most men. It has a distinctive odour and may accumulate in the absence of personal hygiene, mixing with exfoliated tissue cells to form an irritating pebble-like calculus. A similar substance is secreted by glands of the clitoris and labia minora.

SNAFU an American abbreviation for 'situation normal: all fucked up.' The expression orginated among soldiers in World War II, and was 'cleaned up' later for civilian use to stand for 'situation normal: all fouled up!

snake phobia an intense, morbid fear of snakes. Evidence from the biblical Garden of Eden, as well as from dreams, fantasies, artistic productions and primitive rituals indicates that the snake represents the penis and fear of snakes symbolizes fear of intercourse. The psychiatric term for snake phobia is ophidiophobia.

snake symbol the representation of a snake as found in dreams, primitive rites, sculptures, and ceramics. The snake is believed to represent the penis as well as fertility.

snatch a slang term for female genitals.

snatch purser a slang term for pimp.

snog a colloquial British term meaning to pet.

snuff movies pornographic films of the worst kind, in which sexual excitement is linked intimately to torture and in which the victim gets actually killed in front of the camera.

S.O.B. an abbreviation for son of a bitch.

social disease a euphemistic expression for venereal, or sexually transmissible, disease.

social hygiene preventive measures for the control of venereal, or sexually transmissible, diseases (also euphemistically known as social diseases), including dissemination of information on these conditions and their social effects as well as promotion of sex education and information on community conditions that serve as a breeding ground for prostitution and other forms of sexual delinquency. The term social hygiene is being replaced by social health, as in the title American Social Health Association.

socialization of sex social customs and characteristics derived from primary male-female differences essential to reproduction. The most prevalent and enduring social differences are those related to functions essential to survival and reproduction—for example, child rearing and homemaking. Beyond these are behaviour patterns characteristic of the particular culture, such as sex hospitality among the Eskimos, partner swapping among suburban 'swingers,' and the various taboos found in restrictive societies.

sodomia Imperfecta a medieval Christian term for 'unnatural' sexual intercourse, particularly anal intercourse among homosexuals. The crime was distinguished from other sexual offences as one that would be handled by ecclesiastical courts rather than civil courts—which were responsible for adultery and similar crimes. In the 12th century, punishment for homosexuality among members of the priesthood included confinement in a monastery.

sodomy a group of sexual variations that are illegal in many jurisdictions, including intercourse of any kind with animals, as well as anal intercourse and mouth-genital contact between human beings. The name is derived from the ancient city of Sodom where corruption was so rampant that it was destroyed, according to the Book of Genesis. A person who practises sodomy is a sodomite.

soft chancre the genital ulcer associated with an infection of *Haemophilus ducreyi*. It begins as a small reddish pimple that fills with pus and becomes a punched-out sore that discharges pus profusely. Unlike the hard chancre, the soft chancre can be quite painful and tends to occur in multiple lesions.

soft media fetish objects that are soft, frilly, or fluffy, such as lingerie. Unlike hard-media objects, soft-media fetish materials can be loose-fitting. While black is a popular colour, soft-media garments can be in other colours, as demonstrated by the colours of garments purchased by men for their wives or girlfriends. Furs are usually considered an example of soft media.

soft-tissue metastases cancers that develop in various body organs and tissues, excluding bones, as a result of the spread of cancer cells from the prostate gland. The most common sites include the lymph nodes of the lower abdomen, the lymph nodes of the bronchial area, the liver, the lungs, the adrenal glands. Because cancer of the prostate tends to be painless, men generally are unaware of the disease until other organs or body areas have become involved in the spread of cancer cells.

soixante-neut the French term for sixty-nine.

solicitor general a slang term for penis.

somatic sex the sex chromosome complement of the somatic, or body, cells of a persons.

son of a bitch an offensive and vulgar address, with no relation to the literal meaning.

Soranos of Ephesus a Greek physician believed to be one of the first gynaecologists who described abortifacients and contraceptives in detail, maintaining that it is far more advisable not to conceive than to destroy the embryo.

Sorenseen Report a report of a nationwide US survey of young people's sexual activities published in 1973 by the social psychologist Robert C. Sorenson, entitled *Adolescent Sexuality in (Contemporary America.* The study reveals among other things that 75 percent of boys and 60 to 70 percent of girls between 13 and 15 masturbate; and that between the ages of 13 and 19, 59 percent of boys and 45 percent of girls had experienced sexual intercourse.

sororate marriage between a man and two or more sisters (sometimes successively: after the death of the first sister or the discovery that she is infertile). The custom is wide- spread and is often the preferred form of polygyny, as it is in many parts of Africa, in many Native American nations, and in the Caucasus, Papua New Guinea, New Hebrides, northeastern Asia, and the Solomon Islands.

soul kiss another term for 'French kiss.'

spacing of pregnancies the use of birth-control measures such as abstinence and contraception to regulate the period of time between one pregnancy and another. Pregnancies that follow each other too closely have been found to be injurious to the health of both mother and child-for example, it has been found that when births are only 1 year apart the death rate for babies is about 50 percent higher than when births are 2 years apart.

Spanish collar a condition in which the foreskin, or prepuce, becomes too tight, producing irritation of the penis, frequent erections, and painful swelling. The condition can be corrected by circumcision.

Spanish fly a powder known as cantharides made from a species of dried beetles that is native to Franc and Spain. The substance is a powerful irritant that has been used to stimulate the sex, organs, producing priapism in men, but so dangerous that it can be lethal. De Sade was accused of poisoning prostitutes by giving, them the substance as an aphrodisiac.

spanking and sex a term referring to spanking as a form of sexual stimulation. Studies have shown that children can be aroused by spanking—which may be one reason many of them 'invite punishment. The buttocks and anal area are erogenous zones, and this form of stimulation may implant masochistic or sadistic tendencies.

spare a collective male slang term for women available for sexual activity. It is most commonly used in 'a bit of spare,' meaning a woman with no male escort.

spatter one's boots a humorous British euphemism

meaning to urinate-also as *splash one's boots.*

speak Low Genitalese an American slang term meaning to have oral sex.

spectstoring a term introduced by Masters and Johnson to describe the behaviour of an individual who likes to observe his own sexual performance as if he were a spectator. The researchers suggested that the compulsion to rate one's own performance in the sex act is self-defeating because it is assumed that a 'full sexual response does not allow room for the person to simultaneously evaluate the response because the assessment inhibits experiencing the total erotic feeling.

spectrophilia a morbid attraction to ghosts or evil spirits; also, the fantasy, or illusion, of having sexual relations with phantoms. This disorder, or paraphilia, was far more common during the Middle Ages and early modern era than today, particularly in monasteries and nunneries, where it probably arose from extreme sexual repression and possibly from guilt over masturbation or other sexual activity.

speculum an instrument used for examining a body opening, particularly the vagina. A vaginal speculum, sometimes called a bivalve speculum, contains two smooth blades that can be separated by turning a small knob on the handle of the instrument. With the blades open, the examining physician can see rather clearly the inside of the vagina and the cervix of the uterus.

spend a slang term meaning to ejaculate.

spend a penny a British euphemism meaning to urinate.

sperm the spermatozoa; also, the seminal fluid containing spermatozoa.

sperm agglutination the immobilization of sperm because of a blockage of the ductus deferens. The occlusion results in the production of antibodies against the man's own sperm. The antibodies immobilize or agglutinate the sperm so that they lose their motility when ejaculated. The condition can also be the result of orchitis.

sperm analysis another term for semen analysis.

sperm aster a pattern that appears in the newly fertilized ovum characterized by cytoplasm granules radiating from the head of the sperm. Also called aster of fertilization.

spermatemphraxis any obstruction to the normal passage of semen.

spermatic canal the inguinal canal of the male. The term is sometimes used to distinguish the opening front the similar structure in the female.

spermatic-cell arrest a condition in which 'the spermatogenic process of the male reproductive system does not undergo the reduction-division stage leading to production of secondary spermatocytes. This is a common cause of azoospermia.

spermatic cord a cordlike structure composed of connective tissue, blood and lymphatic vessels, and nerves, and containing the ductus deferens. It extends frcm the deep inguinal ring of the abdomen to the upper pole of the testis on each side.

spermatic duct an alternative term for the ductus deferens, or vas deferens.

spermatid an immature form of a spermatozoon in the lining of a seminiferous tubule. It usually appears as a spherical cell embedded in a Sertoli cell, having derived from the division of a secondary spermatocyte. During the spermatid stage, its nucleus evolves into the head of a spermatozoon, the cell protoplasm becomes the middle piece, and the centrioles becomes the tail. The spermatid receives its haploid number of chromosomes in dividing from a secondary spermatocyte.

spermatocelectomy a surgical procedure for removal of a spermatocele, a cystic dilatation of the ducts of the upper part of the epididymis.

spermatocyte an early stage in the development of a spermatozoon from a primitive gamete. A primary spermatocyte derives, from the division and enlargement of a spermatogonium and contains the diploid (46) number of chromosomes. By meiotic division, the primary spermatocyte divides into two secondary spermatocytes, each with the haploid (23) number of chromosomes. In the next division, it becomes two spermatids.

spermatogenesis the process of formation and development of spermatozoa from primordial male germ cells in the walls of the seminiferous tubules through a complex series of mitotic and meiotic cell divisions.

spermatogenic cells one of the two types of cells in the germinal tissue of the seminiferous tubules. The second type of cell is the Sertoli or sustenacular cell.

spermatogonia the basic male germ cells located in the lining of the walls of the seminiferous tubules of the testes. Through repeated mitotic divisions, spermatogonia evolve into primary spermatocytes.

spermatolysin a substance found in the vagina of some women who are hypersensitive to semen or spermatozoa. The substance destroys the spermatozoa.

spermatophobia a morbid fear of semen.

spermatorrhoea a copious emission of semen, which may occur without orgasm. A nocturnal emission may be termed *spermatorrhoea dormientum.* False spermatorrhoea is a form of the condition in which only seminal fluid, without spermatozoa, is discharged.

spermatozoon a single mature male gamete consisting of a conical head, a nucleus, a middle piece of cytoplasm, and a flagellate tail or end piece that helps propel the spermatozoon towards fertilization of an ovum in a fallopian tube.

spermaturia an alternative term for semenuria, or seminuria, indicating the presence of semen or spermatozoa in the urine.

sperm bank a storage depot for frozen sperm to be used in artificial insemination.

sperm cell a spermatozoon or one of its precursors, such as a spermatid.

spermicide any agent that may be used to kill spermatozoa and therefore may serve as a contraceptive. Many spermicides contain one of the nonoxinol chemicals, each of which is identified by a following number indicating its particular molecular structure, such as nonoxinol-10.

sperm life the length of time that a spermatozoon may remain viable after being ejaculated. Studies show that under ideal conditions an ejaculated sperm may live up to 14 days. In the vagina, however, sperm seldom remain viable for more than 2 days. Sperm longevity before ejaculation can be measured in weeks and months, as evidenced by conceptions produced by men who have undergone vasectomies but remain fertile long after the operation.

sperm morphology the shapes and sizes of various spermatozoa in a sample. In fertility studies, the percentage of abnormal spermatozoa forms is considered. At least 80 percent should be within the limits of shapes and sizes considered normal. Particular attention may be paid to the proportions of certain abnormal forms.

sperm-producing tubules an alternative term for the seminiferous tubules of the testis, where primitive spermatogonia are spawned and nurtured until they are ready to enter the epididymal pipeline as mature spermatozoa.

sperm speed the forward progress of spermatozoa after ejaculation. Human spermatozoa have been recorded moving at an average rate of 1.5 millimetres per minute, a speed that is comparable to the speed of a human swimmer when the relative size of a spermtozoon is taken into consideration. At this rate of speed, spermatozoa should be able to travel approximately 1 inch every 15 minutes. Various other species apparently receive help from muscular contractions of the cervix or uterus; for example, spermatozoa of a dog have been found in the fallopian tubes 1 minute after ejaculation. For a rabbit, about 4 hours are required to complete the trip from copulation to the end of the fallopian tube; the timetable for ram sperm is about the same. Human spermatozoa usually reach the 'lover's lane' portion of the fallopian tube within a few hours after ejaculation.

sperm vitality the longevity of spermatozoa in the female reproductive tract. Of the estimated 300 million spermatozoa in a single male ejaculation, it is believed that no more than a few thousand survive for as long as 3 days. By comparison, human sperm have been kept alive outside the body for 2 weeks. Among other animals, experiments indicate rabbit sperm loses its ability to fertilize within 30 hours and is usually dead within 2 days. The sperm of male domestic fowl have been found alive and well in the oviducts of a hen after 3 weeks. Unusual is the bat, which copulates in the autumn even though fertilization does not occur until after hibernation in the following spring.

sphincter a ringlike voluntary or involuntary muscle that surrounds an opening of the body, expanding to open it and contracting to close it as the anal sphincter.

sphincter control the ability to voluntarily open or close the openings of the body that depend upon contraction or relaxation of circular bands of muscle fibres, such as the anal and urinary sphincters, and, in some women, the sphincter cunni. The development of this ability is considered an important step in psychosexual maturation.

sphincter cunni the bulbospongiosus muscle which in the male completely encircles the back of the penis including the corpora cavernosa and corpus spongiosum and in the female surrounds the orifice of the vagina. Also called bulbocavernosus muscle.

spider bite a relatively common cause of oedema of the scrotum. The scrotum tissues are quite sensitive to any inflammatory reaction. The scrotum becomes filled with fluid and greatly swollen, requiring bed rest with the scrotum elevated to help drainage of the lymph vessels and veins.

spinnbarkeit the formation of a stretchable thread of mucus from the uterine cervix, an effect that is possible only at the time of ovulation when the cervix is under the influence of increased oestrogen secretion. The ability of the mucus to be formed into thin strands several inches in length results from a chemical effect on the mucus. It is believed that the chemical change enhances the ability of spermatozoa to move quickly to the cervix along the strands of mucus at the precise time that the woman is at the fertile peak of the menstrual cycle. The spinnbarkeit filaments therefore become a temporary express route to the uterus.

spinster an outmoded and now-insulting term for a woman who remains unmarried beyond the 'usual' age for marriage, and seems unlikely ever to be married. Today many 'spinsters' have an active sex life, and some adopt children or give birth to illegitimate children.

Spirochaeta pallida the Treponema pallidum species of spiral-shaped bacteria that causes syphilis and possibly some nonvenereal forms of spirochaetal infections.

sponge contraceptive a polyurethane-foam sponge designed to be inserted into the vagina as a means of preventing conception, In contrast, to the use of ordinary sea sponges, which dates back to ancient times and is extremely unreliable, today's sponges contain a spermicide that is continually released for about 24 hours Many authorities consider these sponges to be safe and highly reliable.

spontaneous abortion the medical term for miscarriage, or premature expulsion of the foetus when this occur, without intention on the part of the pregnant woman, and without the use of any artificial method. Most spontaneous abortions take place before the third month of foetal life, and are most likely to occur when the mother is below the age 20. Risk of losing the child is about twice as high in a fourth pregnancy as in a first. In many cases the cause is not known, although hormonal imbalance, illness, trauma, malnutrition, or a defective foetus may be factors. A woman who has had a spontaneous abortion can usually conceive again, and have a normal pregnancy.

spontaneous urethral rupture the sudden failure of the wall of the urethra, sometimes occurring at a point previously weakened or damaged by a catheter. The pressure of urine release during routine urination may break through the weak spot, resulting in inflammation of surrounding tissues. Spontaneous urethral rupture also can be a result of obstruction stemming from a stricture in the urethra.

sport an organism that has undergone mutation and has become obviously different in appearance from its parents or ancestors. The term is used in genetics.

sport of Venue a 19th-century euphemism for intercourse.

spousal rape a synonym for marital rape.

spunk a slang term for semen.

squash preparation an assortment of the chromosomes taken from a body tissue cell of a male or female before the chromosomes are arranged in a karyotype. The chromosomes are 'captured' during the metaphase stage of cellular division by the injection of a chemical that freezes the structures in their typical patterns and sizes. The chromosomes are photographed, and the photo images are cut from the print for use in a karyotype.

squeeze technique a method for treating premature ejaculation, preferably under the guidance of a sex therapist. The female partner stimulates erection, then squeezes or pinches the head of the man's penis with her fingers as soon as he signals that ejaculation is about to take place, Repetition of this manoeuvre conditions him to achieve a normal delay in ejaculation.

stag films short films in which sexual acts are explicitly depicted. Generally speaking, these films are not exhibited in standard cinemas but in private showings at clubs and parties. The audience was at one time confined to men, but today women may be included.

standing coitus intercourse with one or both partners in a standing position. Variations include both partners standing face to face (the shorter partner may stand on a stool); the knee-and-elbow position in which the man places his two arms under the women's knees, supporting her on his elbows and raising her as high as his waist; face-to-face with the man raising one of the woman's legs while the other remains on the floor to support her body; face-to-face with the woman clasping her hands behind the man's neck and clasping his waist with her legs; and, most difficult of all, a position in which the man stands while the woman is upside down with her legs around his neck, performing fellatio while he performs curmilingus.

status orgasmus a term sometimes applied to a rapid series of orgasms experienced by some women while enjoying the third stage, or orgasm stage, of the sexual response cycle. Typically, these orgasms are experienced as a single sustained climax followed by a more or less protracted resolution phase.

statutory rape in the USA, sexual intercourse with a female who is below the age of consent.

staying power a slang term for the ability of a man to delay ejaculation after penetration of the vagina until both sex partners are ready for orgasm.

STD abbreviation for sexually transmitted disease.

steatopygia an extreme accumulation of fat in the female buttocks, especially among Hottentots and Bushmen in southern Africa. In these and other cultures, huge buttocks are considered a mark of beauty and sexual attraction.

Steinach, Eugen an Austrian physician who pioneered sex-change medicine in the 1920s. Steinach claimed to have changed the sex of a patient with surgery and hormone injections. Steinach also consulted with psychiatrist Sigmund Freud about the role of sex hormones in certain emotional disorders.

sterility infertility; inability to produce off-spring. Sterility that is voluntary is called facultative sterility. Relative sterility is a form in which fertility is theoretically possible but in which one or more factors such as a low sperm count reduce the chances of normal fertilization. Revocable sterility is a form in which an obstacle to fertility can be removed, as in reconnecting the vas-deferens or fallopian-tube portions previously severed as a means of contraception.

sterilization rendering an individual incapable of reproduction. A female is sterilized by a process of interrupting the sequence of steps necessary to conceive, such as surgical removal of the ovaries, fallopian tubes, or uterus, or a combination of those organs, or by ligating the tubes so that an ovum released during ovulation cannot be fertilized. A male is sterilized usually by surgical vasectomy in which the ductus deferens is severed so that spermatozoa cannot be ejaculated during intercourse. Male sterilization also may be produced by castration, or surgical removal of the testes, as in the treatment for testicular cancer. A vasectomy or tubal ligation can in certain cases be corrected surgically so that fertility may be restored.

steroidogenesis the process whereby steroid hormones, particularly the sex hormones, evolve in biosynthetic steps from cholesterol molecules.

steroids a category of chemical substances that includes the sex hormones. Steroids have in common a specific molecular structure, although they do not all produce the same or similar effects. Besides sex hormones, steroids include cholesterol, vitamin D, bile acids, and toad poisons.

stigma a physical or mental trait that distinguishes an individual from others and is usually considered a mark of disgrace. An unconventional sexual preference or sexual activity may be a stigma in a particular community or culture. The term is also used to refer to a spot on the surface of an ovary that indicates the site of a future rupture of a graafian follicle.

stillbirth birth of a dead child. In contrast to a miscarriage, which usually occurs very early in pregnancy, the stillborn foetus is beyond the sixth month of pregnancy and fully recognizable as a dead baby. Though the cause of a particular stillbirth may be obscure, some of the factors that are commonly involved are immaturity of the foetus, syphilis, protracted labour, water in the lungs, and strangulation by the umbilical cord.

stinginess extreme penuriousness or miserliness. In psychoanalysis, it is a character trait believed to stem from fixation at the anal-retention stage when the child derives pleasure and power from withholding the faeces.

stone baby a foetus that dies within the uterus without being aborted and is instead preserved by a bonelike layer of calcium salts. The calcium shroud presumably develops to protect the mother from the toxic effects of the dead foetus. A stone baby may remain undetected in a uterus for many years. In one recorded case, a stone baby was removed surgically after 61 years in the womb of a woman.

stones a slang term for testicles.

Slopes, Marie Carmichael a British scientist who proclaimed women's right to personal fulfilment and sexual satisfaction in marriage. She opened the first British birth-control clinic in 1921, advocated the use of the diaphragm or Stopes cap for contraception, and founded the Society for Constructive Birth Control. Her books, *Married Love* *and Wise Parenthood*, were widely read and, contributed greatly to the sexual liberation of women.

stop-start technique a two-step sex-therapy method used in overcoming premature ejaculation. In the first step, the man stops 'all' stimulation, whether by himself or by his partner, just as he approaches the moment of inevitable ejaculation. When that moment has passed, he starts again, and by repeating this progress will gradually gain control over the timing of his ejaculation. The same procedure can be followed during masturbation.

storge a Greek term for a form of love that is generally interpreted as synonymous with affection, as distinguished from erotic or passionate love, or philia or agape. Storge is sometimes defined as a nondiscriminating type of love that one may show to parents, children, or pets.

stork a bird invoked in old wives' tales, or in explaining childbirth to young children, as the bringer of babies into the world.

stork bites a fanciful name for pink or purple marks found on the face and scalp of some infants at birth. The lesions, which resemble birthmarks, gradually fade and usually have disappeared by the end of the first year.

straddle injury an injury to the penis, urethra, or adjacent structures as a result of falling astride a hard blunt or sharp object One of the serious effects is a rupture of the urethra at a point behind the scrotum. The corpora cavernosa and corpus spongiosurn are usually damaged at the same time.

straight a colloquial term meaning (a) heterosexual,

or (b) proper, conforming to the norms of the establishment—'square'.

Straight Partners an American organization to help straights who have married homosexuals.

strangulation a type of phimosis that occurs mainly in young boys who insert the penis through a metal ring or other hard metal object, after which swelling occurs so that the penis cannot be withdrawn. If the device is not removed, usually with a jeweller's saw, gangrene can develop, requiring amputation of the affected part of the penis.

streaking the practice of running around in the nude in public places in order to shock others present. Occasionally a means of political protest, it is more often done simply for a dare. Sports matches are popular targets for streakers. It was particularly prevalent in the early 1970s, but it has not entirely died out.

street hustlers teenage practitioners of male homosexual prostitution who solicit clients in the street.

stretch marks a popular term for the lines that appear on the abdomen and other body areas of women as a result of pregnancy. The marks also may be caused by obesity and certain illnesses, such as Cushings syndrome.

streetwalker a euphemism for a prostitute, particularly one who solicits on the streets.

strictures any abnormal narrowing of a passageway, such as the urethra, that can interfere with normal functioning of the reproductive system. Strictures may result from scarring, tears, punctures, or other injuries, such as damage to the lining of the urethra from insertion of a urinary catheter. The symptoms include pain and difficulty in urination and a nonvenereal discharge. The structure can be a cause of impotence. In a woman, a stricture can develop in the urethra, from similar causes such as improper use of a urinary catheter during medical treatment. Strictures also can develop in the fallopian tube or the cervical os, thereby blocking the passage of spermatozoa en route to the fertilization of an ovum. Strictures of the falllopian tubes or cervical os are more easily corrected than strictures of the urethra.

striptease a sexually provocative performance in which women, or in some instances men, parade or dance fully clothed, and then slowly expose more and more of their body by removing one article of clothing after another. Striptease is especially appealing to voyeurs.

stroll an American slang term for street walking, a practice used by some prostitutes to make themselves available to the local male population.

stroma the fibrous framework surrounding the ovaries.

stud a slang term meaning (a) any male (b) a male who is young and carefree, and (c) a male whose masculinity is beyond doubt especially if it is proven through many sexual conquests.

subfecundity a fertility level that is below normal for a female as in relative sterility or one-child sterility, a type of female infertility that follows the birth of the first infant

subincision a form of genital mutilation consisting of a slitting of the underside of the penis with permanent opening of the urethra. It is part of the puberty rites of certain Australian and Fijian societies.

sublimation a psychoanalytical term for the unconscious process of channelling sexual or aggressive drives into acceptable expression, for example, an exhibitionistic urge may gain an approved outlet in ballet training or a voyeuristic impulse may be expressed in the use of a microscope for scientific research.

submission compliance of one individual with the sexual wishes and demands of another person. Some play a passive, submissive role, waiting for their husband or lover to initiate sexual activity. Extreme submission is amplified by the Romans, who subjected female slaves to every form of sexual indignity; and by the practice of erotic bondage and discipline in some areas of society today.

substitute sex partner an especially trained surrogate used in sex therapy.

substitution the replacement of one type of satisfaction with another, as in 'raiding the refrigerator when disappointed in love; also, the replacement of unacceptable impulses with socially acceptable activities, as in cleaning the house from cellar to attic as a substitute for the 'unclean impulse to be promiscuous.

subtotal hysterectomy a hysterectomy that involves removal of the uterus at or above the level of the cervix, the isthmus of the uterus. Also called supracervical hysterectomy.

succubus a medieval term for a demon who assumes the shape of a woman and has intercourse with a sleeping man.

sucking impulse the Impulse to apply suction with the lips, which first appears in early infancy when the nipple is grasped in the feeding process. According to Freud, sucking is the earliest form of autoerotic gratificatiom it later takes the form of thumb sucking and sucking the Partner's tongue, nipples vulva, clitoris, or penis during sexual relations.

sugar daddy an older man who provides financially for a woman, usually in return for sexual favours.

suicidal sex an alternative term for EROTIC HANGING or AUTOEROTIC ASPHYXIA.

sulgenderism the tendency of boys to associate with boys and girls with girl without sexual involvement This occurs Primarily during the 'latency' years before puberty. The term derives from Latin of ones own sex. After puberty, relationships cease to be exclusively with ones own sex.

summa libido the highest point, or summit of erotic pleasure, reached during the orgasmic phase of the sexual response cycle.

superego in psychoanalytical theory, the body of conscious and unconscious principles and value judgments that help control conduct. Popularly known as conscience, the superego stems Primarily from our parents and secondarily from our culture. When its demands are no nut as may happen in our social or sexual life, we usually feel a sense of guilt.

superego anxiety in psychoanalytical theory, an anxiety that is frequently experienced when ethical principles, social codes, or parental behests are violated.

superfecundation fertility that is well above what is considered normal; also, the fertilization of two separate ova released in the same menstrual cycle during separate acts of sexual intercourse with the same male or different males.

superfemale a term sometimes applied to a female born With more than the normal XX complement of female chromosomes, In some rare cases of sex-chromosome aberrations, females have been found with as many as five X chromosomes. Women born with three or more X chromosomes occur at a frequency slightly greater than one per thousand. However, the additional X chromosomes are often associated with mental retardation, sterility, and, despite the term superfemale, under developed female sexual characteristics.

superfoetation the conception of a second foetus by a woman already pregnant as a result of the fertilization of an ovum released in a later ovulation-an extremely rare occurrence.

superincision a form of genital mutilation performed on adolescent boys among the Mangaians and other Polynesian societies as Pad of their puberty rites, The foreskin is pulled over an object called an anvil, the purpose of which is to protect the glans during the incision which runs the entire length of the penis. No anesthetic is used, and there is much bleeding. The boy runs into the sea for relief, shouting, 'Now I am really a man!' The penis is treated with poultices as it heals.

superior-kneeling position an intercourse position in which one partner kneels above the other. Masters and Johnson recommend that the woman use due position if her male partner tends to be impotent. It gives her maximum control over the insertive process, and enables her to avoid pelvic thrustig, which is very demanding for the male. Men suffering from partial impotence find insertion difficult and may low their erection at this point.

supermale a term sometimes applied to a male born with more than the normal complement of male chromosomes, Early study findings suggested that men with XYY chromosome sets were large and aggressive because of the extra male chromosome. However, the first cases were discovered in prison inmates; and further study showed that normal, average men in the general population may also have an extra male chromosome.

supernumerary breasts an alternative term for polymastia.

supernumerary chromosome a chromosome that is in addition to the normal complement of the individual, does not match any of the normal chromosomes for the species, and apparently has little if any effect on the physical appearance of the individual, Supernumerary chromosomes are found occasionally in wild populations of some animals.

supernumerary tube a congenital anomaly consisting of an extra fallopian tube that runs alongside a normal functioning tube. It may or may not be associated with a supernumerary ovary.

superovulate to produce a number of mature ova from the ovary at the same time. This frequently happens as a result of treatment with fertility drugs.

supersex a superfemale or supermale possessing

extra female or male chromosomes. A supersex male would have a complement of 47,XYY, or a total of 47 chromosomes including two Y, male, chromosomes, as compared with the normal 46 chromosome total, including one X and one Y sex chromosome for a male individual. A supersex female would have a chromosome complement of 47,XXX with one extra female, Y, chromosome.

superstraight a latent homosexual who exhibits an antihomosexual attitude as a reaction formation. Thus, a person who persecutes homosexuals may actually be expressing anxiety about his own homosexual feelings.

suprapubic pertaining to a Surgical procedure in which the pelvic cavity is entered through the lower abdomen. The approach is used in some treatments of prostate difficulties, such as obstruction of the urethra. After an incision through the lower abdominal wall, the urinary bladder is opened so that a tumour or other abnormal growth can be removed through the bladder.

suprasellar disease any disorder caused by a rumour or other lesion, including an injury, to the hypothalamus or the stalk connecting the hypothalamus and the pituitary gland. A suprasellar disease may be hypogonadism or precocious puberty. The term suprasellar refers to the location of the hypothalamus, which is above the seller turcica level of the skull, a depression in the sphenoid bone that contains the pituitary gland.

suramin a drug used in Africa to treat protozoal infections and in Europe as an experimental therapy for AIDS infections. Suramin, also called naganol, interferes with the activity of an enzyme that AIDS viruses must use it, order to reproduce.

surface papilloma a type of ovarian tumour in which the growth appears as a mass of tiny warts on the surface of an ovary. It is formed by wildly growing fibrous tissue with multiple branches, each covered with clusters of the minute warts. Untreated, the surface papilloma may continue growing until it fills the pelvic cavity.

surrogate a person who acts in the place of another—for example, a sister, aunt, or uncle who substitutes for the mother or father. In sex therapy, an experienced professional may act as a surrogate partner in helping the patient overcome inhibitions, resistances, and faulty behaviour patterns that stand in the way of satisfactory intercourse.

surrogate mother a woman who takes the place of a sterile wife for the purpose of insemination by the husband. This form of impregnation is unusual. Surrogate mother- hood is the subject of legal dispute as to the rights of the surrogate mother over the child she bears.

surrogate partner a substitute sex partner who has been especially trained to participate in sex therapy.

surrogate therapy treatment of sexual problems through the use of professionally trained and supervised substitute sex partners. Through sympathetic and skilful cooperation, these partners-male or female, as the case may require-help the patient overcome the hindrances to sexual performance, such as tension, anxiety, fear of failure, and lack of confidence, Through a step-by-step procedure, at least one half of male patients suffering from premature ejaculation or impotence, and female patients afflicted with vaginismus or frigidity, can be effectively treated, according to Masters and Johnson, the originators of this technique.

suspensory ligament a strong fibrous triangle of tissue that extends from the linea alba of the belly to the top of the penis, with attachments also to the symphysis pubis.

sustenacular cells the cells of the seminiferous tubules of the testis, which have the function of nurturing the spermatozoa at various stages of their production and maturation.

suttee a Hindu custom in which a widow demonstrated her devotion to her husband by cremating herself on his funeral pyre. The practice was outlawed by the British in 1824.

sweating response the production of a mucoid lubrication fluid directly from the walls of the vaginal barrel and to a lesser extent from Bartholin's glands during the excitement phase of the female sexual response cycle. The biological function of this secretion is to prepare the vagina for entry by the penis.

sweetmeat a slang term for woman.

swing both ways a slang term meaning to be bisexual.

swinging a euphemistic term for partner swapping or mate swapping, though some- times more widely applied to individuals or couples who engage in a wide variety of sexual practices with a wide variety of partners in their search for exciting sexual experiences.

swish a slang term meaning to walk in an effeminate manner, including 'feminine' hip movements. The term is usually applied to the swishy type of male homosexual.

switch hitter an American slang term for a bisexual man or woman.

swive a once-common term meaning to have intercourse. Swive was popular since the 14th century, but by the 18th century it had become almost as vulgar as 'to fuck,' and soon fell into disuse.

Swyer's syndrome a form of mate pseudohermaphroditism in which the individual is genetically a male, with an XY set of chromosomes, but has the internal and external sexual organs of a female. The person is usually raised as a girl, possesses a vagina, uterus, and fallopian tubes, but does not menstruate and fails to develop breasts and other adult female characteristics.

symbiotic marriage a marriage characterized by an extreme degree of mutual dependence, similar to the relationship between mother and infant. In many instances a marital relationship of this kind is based upon neurotic needs, and becomes so close that the partners cannot function without each other.

symbolic masturbation various acts that are believed to substitute for manipulation of the genital organs, such as rubbing the nose, pulling the ear lobes, twisting strands of hair, constantly playing with one's watch or adjusting one's tie.

symphysis pubis the foremost portion of the pubic bone on either side, or more specifically to the joint formed by the meeting of the right and left pubic bones, an area that usually is covered with pubic hair.

symptothermal method a birth-control technique that depends upon a combination of basal-body-temperature monitoring and examination of cervical mucus to determine which days of the menstrual month are

symptothermal method a birth-control technique that depends upon a combination of basal-body-temperature monitoring and examination of cervical mucus to determine which days of the menstrual month are days when intercourse is most likely to result in a pregnancy- Like other birth-control techniques that avoid the use of synthetic hormones, IUD's, condoms, spermicides, and similar unnatural, methods, the symptothermal method requires a great deal of self- motivation and self-discipline and the ability to make accurate observations of physiological changes. Also called the Billings method.

synergic marriage a marriage in which the partners work together and reinforce each other in their effort to achieve common goals and the satisfaction of their individual needs.

synorchidism the complete or partial fusion of both testes.

synoscheos a congenital male abnormality in which the penis is a part of the scrotum.

syphilis a systemic infection caused by the spiral-shaped bacterium *Treponema pallidum* that is usually transmitted by sexual contact. Although the disease has been well known for hundreds of years, the disease organism was not identified until early in the 20th century. For centuries it was known in Europe and Asia as the 'great pox,' which distinguished the lesions from the disease still called 'smallpox.' Because of public-health measures and the development of diagnostic tests and antibiotics, the incidence of primary syphilis has fallen dramatically since the 1940s. But the number of new cases reported is nearly 90,000 per year in the United States, and the true rate is believed to be higher because many cases are treated privately and are not reported. It takes about 3 weeks after a sexual contact with an infected partner for a primary lesion to appear. During the incubation period the concentration of Treponema organisms increases by tens of millions. The initial lesion is a chancre, a painless pimple that quickly erodes into an ulcer In heterosexual men, the chancre is usually on the penis. In homosexual men, it is usually on the genitalia, in the mouth, or the anal canal. In women, the chancre may appear on the labia or cervix. Lymph glands in the area of the chancre become firm and swollen within a week. The chancre heals within 2 to 12 weeks, but the lymph-gland effects persist. Second- lesions can appear before the chancre heals or several months later. The lesions appear as a skin rash or pink-to-red macules or pimples, some of which may contain pus. The skin lesions may pop up anywhere from the soles of the feet to the scalp. The lesions may be accompanied by fever, loss of appetite, weight loss, and general discomfort. Headaches are common, and the person may experience neuritis and visual problems. After the first 2 years, a syphilis infection may follow a number of courses, but some 50 percent of those untreated are likely to develop inflammation of the aorta and other large blood vessels, or neurosyphilis leading to paralysis or other debilitating physical damage and mental degeneration. The term syphilis comes from the thus infected hero of a 16th-century play by Girolamo Fracastero, a shepherd named Syphilis.

syphilis innocentum a syphilis infection that was acquired by accidental contact with the disease organism rather than through intercourse.

syphilitic adenopathy a disease of the lymph glands resulting from an infection of syphilis. The lymph glands in the area of the original syphilis lesion, whether inguinal cervical, or occurring elsewhere, become swollen and hard. The symptom commonly persists is for some time after the primary syphilis lesion has disappeared.

syphilitic arteriosclerosis a degenerative condition of the arteries, marked by a loss of elasticity of the artery walls, resulting from syphilis.

syphilitic chancre a hard chancre that develops at the site of contact with a person infected with *Treponema pallidum* spirochaetes, particularly during the stage in which the disease organisms are multiplying rapidly in an exposed sore. The point of contact is usually an area of the genitals or mouth. Over a period of about a week, the initial lesion, a painless pimple, evolves into an ulcer-the hard chancre.

syphilitic conjunctivitis a form of conjunctivitis caused by an infection of syphilis and characterized by a variety of lesions of the eye, ranging from conjunctival chancres to gummas.

syphilitic vitiligo an acquired loss of skin pigmentation, especially around the neck, that is a sign of a second stage of syphilis. Also called vitiligo acquisita.

syphilization the development of a relative immunity to syphilis. According to some authorities, repeated exposure to syphilis over several generations in a community may lead to a relative immunity to the disease. There also have been some serious attempts to develop immunity to syphilis by inoculation with the disease organism, *Treponema pallidum.*

syphiloma a tumour that is related to a syphilis infection, such as a gumma.

syphilophobia a morbid fear of syphilis.

sypho an Australian colloquialism for syphilis.

T

taboo a Polynesian term for an object, act, word, gesture, or person that is prohibited by social custom or religious belief in a particular society. Freud describes a taboo as follows: On the one hand it means to us sacred, consecrated; but on the other hand it means uncanny, dangerous, forbidden, and unclean. Taboo examples are father-daughter-incest taboo, mother-son-incest taboo, and virginity taboo.

tactile stimulation sexual stimulation through the sense of touch during the state of foreplay preceding intercourse. A large proportion of the activities of both partners are tactile, including handholding and kissing and caressing any or all parts of the body, with special attention to the breasts and nipples, and to the buttocks, inner thighs, and genital organs. Licking, sucking, and biting are all tactile, as are tight embraces in which arms and legs are intertwined. All these tactile stimuli increase sexual excitement and prepare the way for intromission.

Tahitians inhabitants of Tahiti, one of the Society Islands in the South Pacific. The island has been called a 'sexual paradise,' based largely on the oft-quoted tale that Tahitian girls would swim out to passing boats in the nude offering themselves to the sailors. That reputation was perpetuated for a time by a religious group known as the Arioi Society, whose members worshipped the goddess of fertility by travelling from island to island as dancers, singers, and sexual exhibitionists. Today there is probably less promiscuity among Tahitians, because of colonialization, but other sexual customs have developed, such as institutionalized transvestites, called Mahu, who act as servants in the chiefs household and frequently enter into homosexual relations with non-transvestite men.

tail a Shakespearean euphemism for (a) the vagina, (b) the penis, and (c) the buttocks. These meanings are still current in slang use, as well as the further meaning of tail as (d) sexual intercourse.

tail dater an American term referring to a system for meeting persons of the opposite sex by obtaining their identity through the registration number of their car. The technique was introduced in southern California where several commercial dating services provide bumper or windowstickers for men or women who, for a fee, supply their names and telephone numbers to be made available to tail daters.

taint an American slang term for the perineum, the area between the anus and the scrotum of a male or between the anus and the vagina of the female—taint because it ain't the one or the other.

take it from behind a slang term meaning to be the passive partner in anal intercourse.

take the sheet a homosexual slang term meaning to be the passive partner in anal intercourse.

talent a collective informal term for the sexually attractive woman especially in the phrase eyeing up the local talent.

tampon a roll of cellulose material designed to absorb the menstrual flow when inserted into the vagina.

Tantric love rite a Hindu sexual rite in which there is a gradual progression of physical and spiritual activities culminating in orgasm. The rite begins with enhancement of the environment with flowers, fruit, incense, music, and candlelight; next come bathing, then oiling and massaging each other, a period of meditation and alternate-nostril breathing, followed by humming a Mantra diving which both partners envisage themselves as Shiva and Shakti, the Supreme Couple. The woman then places herself to the right of the man, and the man proceeds to kiss and stroke her entire body, from toes to head and back again. She then slowly arouses her male partner with her hands and lips in a similar order. Finally, the woman moves to the left of the man for the last stage of sexual fulfilment, in which various prearranged intercourse positions are employed until each of them experiences the transcendental power of love during the climax.

taphophilia a morbid attraction for cemeteries. The term is related to necromania and necrophilia.

tart an obsolescent colloquial term for Prostitute.

tattooing the tattoo-marking of various parts of the body—as for the purpose of enhancing physical attraction and sex appeal. The designs usually express sexual symbolism— for example, snakes, tigers, daggers, or the name of the loved one—and are applied to arms, legs, buttocks, breasts, back, and even the sex organs themselves, Tattoos are prevalent in the United States and Britain, but also in Japan, Africa and Oceania.

T-Cell a lymphocyte that is influenced in some way by the thymus gland, usually by passing through the thymus as it circulates through the body. Various kinds of T-cells can suppress or stimulate antibody production in responding to infectious organ- isms and the formation of tumours, and are capable of destroying some cells. T-cells are involved in natural resistance to sexually transmissible diseases, but in a case of AIDS may be overwhelmed by the infection.

T-cell helper depletion a diagnostic factor in cases of AIDS. Because the HTLV-III virus destroys the helper T-cells that ordinarily engulf and devour microorganisms in the body, the human system gradually loses the battle as its T-cells are depleted.

tear-drop prosthesis a female breast implant that produces the contour of a normal pendulous breast. It is recommended for women with abnormally small breasts and a minimum of 'feminine contour' to the rest of the body.

tearoom trade an American Slang term for male homosexual activity that is based in public lavatories, where a sexual encounter may be conducted in a cubicle.

teasing in sexual behaviour, deliberate acts designed to provoke sexual interest or suggest availability for sexual activity. Teasing ranges from wearing revealing clothes to smiling and flirting, touching, kissing, and sex play short of intercourse. A vulgar slang term for a woman who keeps men dangling in this manner is 'cock-tease' or 'cock teaser'.

teddy-bear syndrome the tendency to form attachments in order to ensure a childlike emotional security rather than on the basis of the sort of compatibility appropriate to an adult relationship. It is often cited as a major reason for the breakdown of many marriages.

teenage pregnancy pregnancy that occurs in females under the age of 20, for whom the majority of births would, be out of wedlock and presumably unintended. In 1985, the United States led nearly all developed nations of the world in teenage pregnancies, abortions, and births The maximum difference in birthrates between the United States and other countries occurred among girls under the age of 15. The United States also was the only country where teenage pregnancy was increasing. The rate of pregnancies among girls 15 to 19 years of age was 96 per 1,000, compared with 14 per 1,000 in the Netherlands, 35 per 1,000 in Sweden. 43 per 1,000 in France, 44 per 1,000 in Canada, and 45 per 1,000 it, England and Wales. The US rate of abortions among teenagers ranged from about 10 per 1,000 at the age of 15 to over 60 per 1,000 at the age of 18.

teenage runaways teenage boys and girls who run away, usually to the 'big city', as a gesture of independence or an escape from an unhappy home or school situation. Many of them can be enticed into prostitution by pimps or the equivalent because of a desperate need for money and someone to care for them-and because they are unaware of the consequences of their sexual activities in terms of disease, drugs, beatings, involvement with the law, and, in general, a sordid life.

teenage sex the introduction of persons to sexual experience before adulthood.

teenybopper a slang term for a female teenager, especially one who identifies with the counter-culture.

telegony the erroneous theory that a 'previous sire' exerts an influence on a later conception. As applied to humans, the theory holds that the offspring of a second husband might be affected by the wife's previous impregnation by her first husband, or simply by having had intercourse with him. However, any resemblance between the child and the first husband has to be regarded as purely coincidental. In the case of animals, the theory gains superficial credence from observations of female dogs, but here the resemblances can probably be explained from the fact that they remain in heat for several days ;d ay mate with several males, making it possible to have a litter in which one or more Puppies appear-falsely-to be a carryover from previous matings.

telephone scatalogia a psychosexual disorder in which a man achieves sexual gratification by making obscene, provocative telephone calls, usuallv to women chosen at random.

temperature eroticism the erotic pleasure of feeling warmth, especially being 'hot' as an accompaniment of sexual desire, fantasy, or activity. The immediate cause is probably increased flow of blood during sexual excitement, and the ultimate cause is the pleasure of warmth experienced when the individual was cuddled by the mother.

temple prostitution another term for sacred prostitution.

temptation the act of tempting, or a thing that tempts, especially into doing something one should not do.

tenderness feelings of warmth, closeness, affection, and caring associated with gentle expressions of love such as stroking, hugging, cuddling and kissing.

tenting effect a term applied to the dilatation of the inner end of the vagina during the plateau phase. It is during this phase that full vaginal expansion occurs.

teratocarcinoma a tumour, such as a testicular tumour, that contains trophoblastic or other embryonic tissues. Teratocarcinomas account for more than one third of all testicular cancers.

teratogen any agent, such as a chemical, virus, or radiation, that can cause foetal malformations or diseases. A teratogen usually disrupts some stage of normal development in an embryo or foetus, with the damage occurring in the first trimester. The classic teratogen, thalidomide, a tranquilizer, disrupts the normal development of arms and legs of a foetus if the mother takes the drug during the fourth week of a pregnancy, when the embryonic arm and leg buds first appear. Hearing and vision, which also first appear then, may be affected as well.

teratological effect a malformation found in a newborn infant that was probably induced by exposure of the mother to a teratogen during the early weeks of the pregnancy and which cannot be attributed to a genetic defect or injury inflicted during labour. Teratological effects may include abnormal vision, hearing deficits, mental retardation, and missing body parts.

teratomatous rest a turnout that evolves from misplaced embryonic tissue and secretes large quantities of chorionic gonadotropin hormone. The effect is sexual precocity, particularly in the male who may show true sexual maturity in childhood. How ever, the tumour is cancerous and usually spreads throughout the body before the cause of the sexual precocity can be corrected.

teratophobia a morbid fear of monsters; also, fear of giving birth to a monstrously deformed or disfigured child.

terebinth a member of the turpentine tree family, one variety of which is the source of an aromatic resin called mastic. Mastic is mixed with salep, a starch made from dried orchid tubers, to produce an alleged aphrodisiac used in India.

term the end of the normal gestation period of between 38 and 42 weeks. The word may refer to the infant born alive during the span of 38 to 42 weeks. An infant born before the 38th week is described as preterm, and one born after the 42nd week may be called postterm.

tertiary sex characteristics a term sometimes applied to personality characteristics of the sexes. These characteristics are now being questioned, but many people associate masculinity with greater physical confidence and endurance, aggressiveness, emotional self-control, and economic competitiveness; and femininity with greater altruism, tenderness, emotionality, and interest in child rearing and homemaking.

testicular agenesis a congenital absence of normal testicular tissue in a male, resulting in a lack of secondary male sexual characteristics. The individual possesses vestigial wolffian ducts terminating in nodules that represent primitive testes that failed to develop normally.

testicular atrophy a loss of function and degeneration of a testis because of disease or injury. Atrophy of a testis may result from an interruption of the blood supply, an infection such as syphilis, the mumps, or filariasis. Congenital syphilis can be the cause of a condition known as 'pigeon's-egg testicle', which may appear large but defective. Interruption of the blood supply, which can occur during surgery, may cause the testis to become both small and functionless.

testicular biopsy a method of obtaining a small sampled a male testicle for study of possible causes of infertility or other problems. A local anesthetic is used to deaden the feeling of the testes, and a small incision is made until the tunica albuginea is visible. Unless there is evidence of a problem elsewhere, such as the vas deferens, a sample of a single testis is usually representative of the condition of the general contents of the scrotum. The single testis sample should show the condition of the Sertoli cells, seminiferous tubules, and other structures. The biopsy is usually coordinated with a semen analysis. The scrotal incision can in most cases be sealed with a couple of sutures after the biopsy sample is taken.

testicular cord an alternative term for spermatic cord.

testicular elevation the involuntary lifting of the testes within the scrotum during excitement. The lifting of the testes, by automatic action of the muscle fibres within the scrotum, is a necessary step towards male orgasm.

testicular failure any dysfunction of the various parts of the testes, resulting in infertility. Causes can include failure of the interstitial cells to produce testosterone, blockage of the vas deferens, or a similar disorder.

testicular feminization an abnormal condition in which a male has the normal complement of an XY set of chromosomes but his body fails to respond to the stimulation of androgenic hormones. As a result, he may develop some feminine characteristics.

testicular tumour a cause of sexual precocity in boys, The features usually are unique in that the child may have pubic hair and an enlarged penis, because of male-sex-hormone production by the testicular tumour, but only one testis is involved. Thus, the scrotum on the side containing the tumour may appear mature, but the testis on the unaffected side remains infantile. The asymmetry of the testicles is a diagnostic sign of the cause of the apparent sexual maturity.

testis the male gonad, which is suspended in the scrotum by the spermatic cord. In foetal life, the testes are located in the abdominal cavity and normally descend into the scrotum before birth, becoming covered in their passage through the inguinal canal with various layers of muscle and connective tissue. The layers include fibres of the cremasteric muscle, and internal and external spermatic fascia, and the tunica vaginalis. Blood vessels and nerves are found in the tissue layers surrounding each testis. The tunica vaginalis is a membrane pouch derived from tissues of the peritoneum, which covers the visceral organs. The tunica vaginalis actually forms in the scrotum before the arrival of the testes from their prenatal location in the abdomen. Each testis contains hundreds of coneshaped lobules—experts differ on the precise number-which in turn contain the seminiferous tubules in which the spermatozoa are produced. The tubules are supported by the interstitial cells which are the source of the male sex hormone testosterone. The lobules have openings that merge as they approach the ductus deferens so that the mature spermatozoa leave the seminiferous tubules by one of the several dozen relatively large ducts feeding into the head of the epididymis. Although each testis is about 1.5 inches long, the left testicle may appear larger because it usually hangs lower.

testis cords the embryonic structure of the male reproductive system that will evolve into the seminiferous tubules.

testolactone an oestrogen inhibitor administered to infertile men whose low sperm count is associated with excessive levels of the female sex hormone.

testosterone the male sex hormone secreted by the interstitial cells of the testis. It is the most potent of all the natural male sex hormones. Variations of the hormone include ethinyl testosterone, which has some of the pharmacological activity of the female sex hormone progesterone; methyl testosterone, a derivative that can be administered orally; testosterone phenylpropionate, and testosterone propionate, a long-acting version of the hormone that can be administered by injection.

testosterone cypionate an injectable form of testosterone supplement for men with sexual dysfunction resulting front abnormally low levels of the male sex hormone. Injection every 3 to 4 weeks reportedly restores potency in many cases of impotence.

testosterone deprivation the effects of castration of the male, whose testosterone hormone is produced in the testes. The effect is observed in birds and other animals, in addition to male humans.

test-tube baby an infant whose conception was produced outside the human body. A test-tube baby is conceived by fertilizing an ovum extracted from the woman with spermatozoa obtained from the man under carefully controlled conditions in a laboratory dish. The fertilized ovum is then implanted in the uterus of the woman.

TFR abbreviation for total fertility rate.

Thai beads an alternative name for vaginal balls.

thalidomide a tranquilizer developed in Germany in 1953 and marketed as a 'safe' sedative. In animal tests it was found that the drug had virtually no toxic effects in massive doses and therefore would be a suitable substitute for barbiturates because it would be virtually impossible for a patient to take a lethal overdose. In 1960, however, it was discovered that pregnant women who took thalidomide were delivered of deformed children with a variety of defects. The most common birth defect was phocomelia, or arms and legs that were extremely short or with Parts missing. In retrospective research, it was found that thousands of women with children so afflicted had taken doses of thalidomide during the fourth week of pregnancy, when the embryonic limb buds were forming. Those who took the drug on days when the eyes or ears were forming gave birth to infants with visual or hearing difficulties. Thalidomide was taken off the market. One important test that had not been performed on the drug was one that would demonstrate the safety of thalidomide during pregnancy. Since the thalidomide tragedy, women have been advised to use extreme caution in taking any drug during pregnancy because medical studies now indicate that many drugs, including alcohol, can cause birth defects,

theca externa a layer of thick, dense connective tissue fibres that forms an outer protective layer around the ovarian follicle. It is adjacent to the theca interna layer, with which it forms a double-layered envelope.

theca interna a layer of tissue cells round the ovarian follicle. It is rich with blood capillaries and lymph vessels interspersed with connective tissue. After the rupture of the follicle releasing the ovum, the theca interna provides the capillaries that support the formation of the corpus luteum..

thecoma a functioning tumour of the ovary that secretes female sex hormones, The tumour is generally found in a postmenopausal woman. It causes irregular menstrual bleeding, breast enlargement, and increased sex drive.

thelalgia a pain experienced in the breast nipple.

thelarche a form of premature puberty in which the female breasts develop in childhood. The cause is usually benign and not the effect of a tumour or other serious disorder.

thelasis a medical term for suckling, or breast feeding.

thelerethism an erection of the nipple as a result of stimulation, as in sexual foreplay, which causes contraction of the muscle fibres of the nipple.

thelitis an inflammation of the breast nipple.

thelybiast the nucleus of a zygote, or fertilized ovum.

thelygenic pertaining to a pattern of giving birth only to female offspring.

thelygonia the production of ova containing only the female (X) sex chromosome. Technically, the term applies to all ova because only the male gametes contain the male, or Y, chromosome.

thelymania an obsolete term for satyriasis.

thelyplasm the portion of a gamete, male or female, that contains the female (X) sex chromosome material.

theoretical failure rate the failure rate of a contraceptive under hypothetical conditions in which nothing goes wrong.

theory of ovum viability the concept that the survival of an individual is related to the viability of the fertilized egg from which he or she develops. The theory is based on experiments with nonhuman mammals in which viability varied according to the amount of time elapsing between ovulation and fertilization of the ovum. Extrapolated to humans, the theory suggests that—excluding environmental factors such as accidents—the quality of the egg cell at fertilization influences the survival of the person.

therapeutic abortion an induced abortion performed to protect the life or physical or mental health of the mother. A therapeutic abortion also might be performed if prenatal evidence indicates that the foetus if born would suffer a severe physical or mental handicap.

therapeutic lovemaking a term referring to Oriental sexual practices based on the Taoist and Tantric doctrine that specific coital postures and rhythms can have a healing effect aphrodisiacs by enabling the body to correct imbalances; for example, some positions enhance circulation of the blood, and others strengthen the bones, rest the spirit, increase the production of marrow, or adjust the whole system, Each of these benefits is believed to be achieved not only by its special 'love posture', but by a specific number of 'strokes of love' by the man, as well as a specific amount of daily practice.

thigh sandwich another term for femoral intercourse.

third sex a mythological tribe living north of the Black Sea who were reputed to be ambisexual. Writings of Plato and Herodotus referred to the tribe, and Plato suggested that the third-sex people eventually died out.

Today, the term may be applied to homo-sexuals when viewed as a sex that is separate and distinct from male or female.

Thongs an agricultural society in Mozambique, organized along polygynous lines, with the sororal type preferred. In this society, kissing is regarded as revolting because of the contact with another person's saliva. Elongated labia minora are considered sexually exciting, and attempts are made to stretch them. Ritual copulation is commonly practised, and widows are required to perform ritual intercourse to cleanse themselves of the spirit of the dead husband; and the headman must have ritual intercourse with his principal wife on the site chosen for a new village.

three-inch fool a Shakesperean term for a man with

a short penis, as in *The Taming of the Shrew* Curtis: Away, you three-inch fool!... Grumio: Am I but three inches? Why, thy horn is a foot, and so long am I at the least.'

thrush a disease of the mucous membranes characterized by white patches, or plaques, in die mouth and vagina, and caused by infection by a fungus, Candida albicans.

thyme a small grey-green shrub that has been the source of medicines and food flavourings since at least the days of Theophrastus, in the 4th century B.C. One of its virtues was said to be its aphrodisiac quality. It also was grown as a plant that attracted honey bees, and honey was always an ingredient of

Tikopia inhabitants of small island in the Pacific Ocean east of the Solomons. Their characteristic sexual customs include coitus interrupters as a means of birth control; adoption of a side-by-side facing position during intercourse; a taboo among males against touching their own genitals or those of their female partners and the use of bananas and roots are dildos.

timing of intercourse preferred times for intercourse. In Western cultures most couples make love during the quiet of the night, though fatigue may interfere with full pleasure if the hour is late. For the sake of variety, they may also change the time to the morning or midday, with an occasional spontaneous 'quickie' at other times, especially on holiday.

tines cruris a ringworm infection of the genital area caused by any of several fungal organisms, including *Epidermophyton floccosom, Trichophyton* *interdigitate,* or *Trichophyton rubrum.* The infection is named after its location, being derived from the Latin crus which is sometimes used to refer to the genital area of the leg or thigh.

tinkle a British euphemism for urination, used particularly in the phrase 'have a tinkle'.

titillatione mammarum a Latin term for coitus intra mammas, once used by prostitutes who specialized in that form of sexual activity and employed the term in advertising their availability.

tits a vulgar slang term for the female breasts. The term, in use for at least 300 years.

tits man a man who is attracted by the female breasts as primary turn-on.

titties a colloquial term for the female breasts.

T.L.C. a common abbreviation for tender loving care.

T-mycopiasma a type of bacteria responsible for a genital tract disease called ureaplasma urealyticum. A related species, *Fmycoplasma,* is believed responsible for many cases of infertility. It has been found in the cervical mucus of infertile women and on the middle piece of the spermatozoa of infertile men.

tobacco stains brown endometrial cysts that are found on the peritoneal membranes of the pelvis. They are caused by the presence of misplaced endometrial tissue, which normally lines the uterus. They are generally noncancerous and cause few if any symptoms. But like endometrial tissue elsewhere, they are under the influence of female sex hormones and react to menstrual cycles like the endometrium of the uterus.

tocoergometry a measurement of the expulsive force of the uterus in childbirth.

tocomania a mental disturbance that sometimes follows childbirth

tocopherol the generic chemical name for vitamin E, an essential nutrient in maintaining a normal pregnancy. Tocopheryl acetate is used in the treatment of habitual abortion. Because of its role in reproduction, it was given its chemical name at the time the substance was first isolated, in 1936.

tocophobia a morbid dread of childbirth.

Todas buffalo herders of southern India whose society is organized along polyandrous lines, usually of the fraternal type, with brothers sharing the same wife. Wives may also have several officially recognized lovers, just as men in other societies have several concubines. In selecting these lovers, one of the major qualifications is strength and skill, especially in catching buffalo for ritual feasts.

toles d'abattage the cheapest kind of mass brothels in Paris in the mid-19th century. It appears that tables were used instead of beds.

tom a British slang term for prostitute.

tomboy a girl who behaves in a manner commonly associated with boys, preferring rough-and-tumble play and the company of boys to pursuits and companions that are ordinarily considered feminine. Such girls are usually going through a stage of rebellion against the restrictions involved in being a 'little lady', as expected in many homes and schools. They usually outgrow their tomboy tendencies, and a few become female homosexuals.

tongue kiss another term for 'French kiss'.

tool a slang term for penis.

tooth alteration filing, blackening, reddening, drilling, pulling, or knocking out teeth for purposes of enhancing sexual attractiveness. These practices are not uncommon among some African societies and Australian aborigines, especially in connection with initiation ceremonies.

topless a colloquial term meaning (a) bare-breasted, especially when referring to dancers, waitresses, and other women in service or entertainment functions, (b) featuring such women, when referring to restaurants, nightclubs, and other places serving the public or (c) tailored in such a way that the breasts are exposed, when referring to a garment. The term is also used as a noun in American English, as in 'She works as a topless,' 'Let's go to a topless,' or 'All her toplesses were designed in Paris.'

topless radio in American English meaning a phone-in programme in which callers can air their sexual problems, and *toPless* TV is a programme that may feature a topless or entirely nude hostess, sometimes with a nude male, and which is usually, but not always, a phone-in show.

top man the active male homosexual partner in anal intercourse—the opposite of the 'bottom man'.

topos a euphemism for lavatory in the 19th century.

TORCH an acronym for remembering the types of infectious organisms that can cause congenital defects in an embryo or foetus. The initials stand for Toxoplasmosis, Other, Rubella, Cytomegalovirus, and Herpes Simplex. The 'other' is generally a euphemism for syphilis.

torsion of the testicle an abnormal rotation of a testicle, resulting in interruption of the blood supply. The condition must be corrected by surgical incision into the scrotum to straighten the spermatic cord. If not corrected early, the interrupted blood flow can result in gangrene, requiring castration to save the life of the man.

TOSOS abbreviation for The Other Side Of Silence, a U.S. homosexual group founded by the playwright Doric Wilson. The term may also refer to the homosexual community in general.

toss off a British slang term meaning to masturbate.

total fertility rate (TFR) the average number of children that would be born alive to a woman during her lifetime if she conformed to an age-specific fertility rate of a given year for her entire childbearing span of life. Unlike the crude birthrate, the TFR is independent of the age structure of a population.

total hysterectomy the removal of the entire uterus, usually through an abdominal wall incision, but sometimes vaginally. The total hysterectomy removes the cervix as well as the body of the uterus, as compared with the subtotal hysterectorny, in which the cervix remains after the body of the uterus is excised.

totem an animal, plant, or natural force such as rain that is revered as the tribal ancestor, symbol, tutelary spirit, or protector of a clan Members of the clan are forbidden to destroy the totem and often may riot have Sexual relations with each other—which Freud interpreted in terms of prevention of incest.

touching tactile contact with another person as a

way of expressing affection or as a means of stimulating erogenous zones during sexual foreplay.

touch up a slang term meaning to touch someone in a sexually sensitive place as a form of furtive sexual advance. For example, a man trying to put his hand up a woman's skirt might be said to be 'touching her up'.

Tourette's syndrome a lifelong disorder starting in childhood, characterized by episodes of involuntary muscle spasms in various parts of the body, vocal tics such as barks, yelps, grunts, and an uncontrollable urge to utter obscenities. The condition was first described by the French physician Georges Gilles de la Tourette, in 1885.

toxaemia of pregnancy any of a series of conditions that may affect a pregnant Woman, such as eclampsia, preeclampsia, gestational hypertension, gestational oedema, gestational proteinuria, or hyperemesis gravidarum.

toxic-shock syndrome (TSS) a combination of symptoms of fever, headache, confusion, vomiting, diarrhoea, and rapidly falling blood pressure caused by an infection of *Staphylococcus aureus*, a bacterium commonly found on the skin and the lining of the genitals. An outbreak of 850 cases of the disease in the USA in 1980 was attributed to the use by some women of super absorbent menstrual tampons. The effects were caused by a toxin produced by the bacterium.

toy boy a derogatory term for a woman's younger male lover. It usually carries the implication that the woman is providing for the man financially, and that he is regarded as little more than a sex object.

TPAL letters used in a system of classifying women

who have been pregnant or have home children. The letters indicate the total number of pregnancies, premature infants, abortions, and number of living children.

transcervical uterine aspiration the removal of fluid, products of conception, or abnormal endometrial tissue by suction. The procedure is commonly used in firstrimester abortions, a technique sometimes identified as vacuum curettage. The cervix is dilated approximately 1 millimetre per week of gestation, and a vacuum tip of about the same diameter is inserted and rotated around the uterine cavity. A local anaesthetic is used, and the procedure usually lasts less than 3 minutes.

transference love a Freudian term for feelings of strong affection and attachment experienced by the patient towards the analyst during the process of therapy. Because psychoanalysis involves the transference, or 'projection,' of unconscious feelings originally directed towards the parents, and the process of 'working through' these feelings, the patient temporarily directs feelings of love towards the analyst. This is an artifact of the process, because it is a reenactment of infantile feelings unrelated to the character or even the sex of the analyst as a person.

transgenderism a gender-identity disorder in which a person strongly identifies with the opposite sex and may cross-dress, yet does not wish to undergo sex-change surgery. The confusion of sex roles usually sterns from a failure of one or both parents to provide adequate sex-role models.

transitional double standard a variation in the traditional or orthodox double-standard concept regarding premarital sex. While the traditional double standard accepts premarital sex for males but not for females, transitional double-standard rules accept the notion that premarital sex for females is acceptable if they are in love or engaged.

transsexualism a gender identity disorder characterized by a persistent sense of discomfort and inappropriateness with ones anatomical sex, as well as an obsessive need to change one's sex organs and live and dress as a member of the other sex. According to the American Psychiatric Association, the diagnosis is made only if the condition has been continuous for at least 2 years and does riot stem from other mental disorders, such as schizophrenia, and is not associated with physical intersex or genetic abnormality.

transurethral referring to a method of examining and treating disorders of the prostrate gland through the urethra. Electroscopic instruments are inserted through the urethral opening at the end of the penis: through the penile and other segments of the urethra, and into the prostate gland and bladder, if necessary. The lighted instruments allow the surgeon to see into the prostate and manipulate devices within the shaft of the instrument for cutting away bits of offending tissue.

transverse birth a 'presentation' occurring once in 200 births, in which the foetus lies crosswise with the arm, shoulder or hand entering the birth canal first. During labour the foetus must be turned, or a caesarean section may be indicated.

transvestism a psychosexual disorder usually characterized by a persistent, often compulsive, urge to wear clothes of the opposite sex as a means of achieving sexual excitement. Cross-dressing, as it is also called, is usually observed among basically heterosexual males whose sexual experience with women is limited, and who may have occasionally engaged in homosexual acts. In many cases their mothers dressed them as girls in childhood because their mother wanted a girl child. In some instances cross-dressing was used as a petticoat punishment.

traumatic evulsion an injury to the male genitalia in which the skin of the scrotum and occasionally the penis is tom away in an accident involving powerful machinery. Traumatic avulsion is a hazard of mechanized farming. The mishap leaves exposed the testicles, which must be surgically reimplanted under the skin of the thigh unless enough skin remains to generate a new scrotum. A skin graft may be needed to speed the healing of the scrotum.

traumatic epididymitis a form of epididymitis that often develops after strenuous physical activity in a young man. It is believed to result from a backflow of urine or prostate secretion from the prostatic portion of the urethra during physical effort, rather than from direct injury to the epididymal tissues.

travail an archaic term for labour pains.

treatment of impotence a therapeutic process in which the primary objective is that of overcoming the 'fear-of-failure' factor in impotence. The therapy requires the active participation of the sexual partner and the creation of an atmosphere in which the male does not feel any pressure to perform, but instead is allowed to relax and enjoy bodycontact pleasures and the emotional interaction of lovemaking, The process may involve stimulating the penis to an erection several times without requiring coitus.

trial marriage an informal marriage arrangement in

which a couple agree to a trial period in which they live together and test their relationship more deeply and comprehensively than is possible during the courting process. They also try to resolve any difficulties they encounter and thereby reduce the possibility of divorce after actual marriage. They usually agree not to have children during the trial period.

tribadism a lesbian practice in which one partner lies on top of the other and simulates coitus by rubbing the genitals together. The partner who plays the 'male' role usually has an especially large clitoris and is called a *tribade*.

TRIC agents a group of chlamydia disease organisms that are strains of *Chlamydia trachomatis* and are responsible for such sexually transmissible disorders as lymphogranuloma venereum, nongonococcal urethitis, pelvic inflammatory disease, and Reiter's syndrome. TRIC agents were originally believed to be viruses but have now been classified as bacteria.

Trichomonas vaginitis an infection of the vaginal tract by a protozoon, *Trichomonas vaginalis*. The effects of the infection include irritation, redness caused by an increased blood flow, swelling of the vulva, and painful intercourse. The condition is also marked by a profuse white discharge, and painful or difficult urination. The Trichomonas organism can be present in the urogenital tract of the male, who may not feet any symptoms although he is capable of reinfecting a female sex partner and should be treated with an antifungal drug, such as metronidazole, at the same time as the female patient.

trichomoniasis an infection by a flagellate protozoon

which often occurs in the human vagina. It may produce a copious white fluid but does not invade the uterus. However, it can be transmitted by sexual contact, causing urethritis in men and vaginitis in women.

trick a slang term for a prostitute's client. The word also is used by homosexual males to distinguish a temporary sex partner from a 'lover'.

trick baby a slang term for a prostitute's child who was fathered by a client.

trilobular pertaining to three lobes, a term that may be applied to the presence of three lobes of prostate tissue that have overgrown the base of the urinary bladder so as to obstruct normal flow of urine. It is one of several variations of prostatic hypertrophy.

trim a slang term for sexual intercourse.

triolism a triadic relationship in which a man engages in sexual relations with a woman and then looks on while she has relation with another man or woman. Similarly, a woman may have intercourse with a man then watches him have relations with another woman or man. The term is also applied by some sexologists to a simultaneous sexual relationship involving three persons; in this case they usually engage in a combination of coitus with oral-genital stimulation.

triorchid a male with three testicles.

triple-X condition a congenital abnormality of some women who have a normal female body but whose body cells contain an extra X, or female sex, chromosome. Fertility is not affected, but the incidence of mental retardation is higher among triple-X females than in the general population. A woman with this condition is called a superfemale, metafemale, or poly-X female.

Trobrianders inhabitants of a Melanesian island in the western Pacific who engage in fishing, gardening, woodcarving, and basket making. Marriage is primarily monogamous although polygyny is permitted. Among their sexual customs are sex expeditions by women as well as men; nose rubbing without kissing; no prostitution, though gifts are given to sex partners; erotic festivals; no punishment for rape; and no attempt at Contraception.

troilism an alternative term for triolism.

TSS abbreviation for toxic shock syndrome.

Tswana a large society living in Botswana in which subsistence is dependent on products of animal husbandry and farming. Marriage is generally polygamous, with the societies form preferred. Sex is performed frequently; in contrast to most primitive societies, foreplay includes sucking and kissing the woman's breasts; co-wives may engage in homosexual acts, especially when the husband is away; and prominent labia minora are considered a major sexual attraction, and from the onset of puberty, girls pull at then and may even resort to killing a bat, burning its wings, and smearing the ashes on cuts made around the labia so that they will become as big as the wings of a bat.

tubal abortion the termination of an ectopic pregnancy within a fallopian tube, Tuba abortions usually occur spontaneously when the pressures of the developing embryo causes, the tube to rupture.

tubal abscess an abscess that can form one or both fallopian tubes of a woman as complication of a gonorrhoeal infection. The condition may be marked by fever, colicky pain, and menstrual irregularity and discomfort.

tubal insufflation a method of testing the patency through the fallopian tubes by injecting a gas, such as carbon dioxide into the uterus. If the gas can pass through the fallopian tubes, a wavy pattern is recorded on an instrument attached to the tube leading into the uterus. If the fallopian tube is obstructed, the pattern will be recorded as a flat curve. The test is used in establishing a cause for infertility.

tubal ligation a surgical sterilization procedure for females in which both fallopian tubes are blocked by applying ligatures, or sutures, that constrict the opening through the tube. Among the various techniques used are the following. In the Irving operation the tubes are ligated, then severed, with one end buried in the muscle tissue of the uterus and the other end buried in a nearby ligament. The Madlener operation involves crushing of the middle section of the tube, which is tied with a nonabsorbable suture material. The Pomeroy operation is one in which the tube is ligated with absorbable material in the middle, then severed. Other techniques are the Uchida operation, the Kroener fimbriectomy procedure, and laparoscopic tubal fulguration. The Madlener, Pomeroy, and Kroener tubal ligations, can be performed through the vagina so that an incision through the abdominal wall is not necessary. Abdominal approaches, such as laparoscopic tubal fulguration, can be relatively simple, requiring only a local anaesthetic. The woman is admitted in the morning and sedated. A small incision is made through the abdomen just below the umbilicus, and the tube is lifted through the incision, to be ligated. The operation itself is usually painless and requires less than a half hour. The woman is observed for several hours for 4 possible side effects or complications and usually returns home the same day. Any abdominal discomfort can usually be treated with aspirin-type drugs.

tubal pregnancy an ectopic pregnancy that occurs in a fallopian tube. It is the most common form of ectopic pregnancy. The tube is likely to rupture as the pregnancy develops, causing the placenta and embryo, or foetus, to drop into the abdominal cavity, where it becomes a tuboabdominal pregnancy. It may also result in a spontaneous abortion.

tubectomy the surgical excision of a fallopian tube.

tuberculosis prostatitis a form of tuberculosis that involves the prostate gland, replacing the normal prostate tissue with fibrous growth and calsification. The condition is generally painless; it is found in about 12 Percent of all terminal cases of tuberculosis.

tuberculous endosalpingitis a disease of the fallopian tubes caused by tuberculosis. The disease is insidious and difficult to diagnose because the woman may experience only menstrual difficulty and a dull pain in the Pelvic area. Meanwhile, the fallopian tube may become inflamed and filled with cheese like pus. The disease is often discovered only during examination to determine a cause of infertility.

tubular testicular adenoma a type of tumour that is found in the gonads of hermaphrodites, the undescended testicles of otherwise normal males, and the ovaries of otherwise normal females who suffer only from amenorrhoea. Because of the frequency of occurrence of the tissue in several genital anomalies, some authorities have attempted to find a correlation. The tissue of the tubular testicular adenoma also is similar to that of the masculinizing-adrenal-gland tumours.

tufting a complication of salpingitis in which the ampullary, or open, end of the fallopian tube is changed so that only a small tuft of fimbriae extends from a closed or partly closed opening. It is, for practical purposes, an obstruction to fertility.

Tukano a Native American society in Brazil whose members believe a pregnant woman should avoid intercourse altogether to keep the number of foetuses from piling up to a point where she may explode. Among the Tukano practices are insertion of a finger into the vagina of girls by an impotent old man as a means of defloration; the requirement that a boy have intercourse with his mother in the presence of his father as part of his coming-of-age ritual; and extreme sexual aggression among women, to a point where seduction of men is a common occurrence and many husbands seek relief by giving their wives anaphrodisiacs.

tumescence a swelling or engorgement that causes enlargement, as in the erection of the penis or clitoris during sexual stimulation.

tunica albuginea a covering of white collagenous fibres that forms a sheath over each of the testes.

Tupinamba a Native American society of hunters and farmers living around Rio de Janeiro. The most prevalent form of marriage is monogamy, though polygyny is permitted. The men wear penis sheaths, and at one time let poisonous animals bite their penises so that they swelled to such a size that women could hardly stand them. Both men and women believe that the woman is simply the greenhouse in which a man's seed grows to become a child, as the anthropologist Edgar Gregersen puts it.

Turkish culture a colloquial term for anal intercourse.

Turner-Ombredanne orchidopexy a surgical procedure for correcting an undescended testicle by suturing it into a compartment on the opposite side of the scrotum, between the septum and the normal testis.

Turner's syndrome a condition in which the gonads fail to develop, usually occurring in females who also manifest a webbing of the neck, short stature, scoliosis, and other physical abnormalities. The cause is a sex-chromosome aberration in which the woman acquires only one X chromosome. She usually has 'streak ovaries' instead of functioning gonads and does not ovulate.

TURP an abbreviation for transurethral resection of the prostate-a procedure to, correct an obstruction of the urinary flow in a male that is caused by an overgrowth of prostategland-tissue. The obstruction is removed via the urethra and by cutting away a portion of the prostate. The procedure is performed with the aid of an endoscope inserted through the urethra for visual control of the resectioning.

tush a colloquial American term for (a) the buttocks or (b) the vagina.

TV an abbreviation sometimes used for transvestite, particularly by members of the transsexual subcultures. A transvestite will use the abbreviation in classified advertisements of underground newspapers to attract persons interested in having sexual contacts with a transvestite.

TV style a slang term for intercourse in 'doggie fashion'. Both can watch TV.

twat a vulgar term for vagina, used since the 17th century.

21-hydroxylase deficiency a congenital defect resulting in the inability of the body's steroid-hormone processes to synthesize desoxycorticosterone from progesterone, one of the steps toward the synthesis of aldosterone hormone. Progesterone is converted instead into 17-ketosteroids, leading to an excessive accumulation of the adrenal hormone. It is the most common congenital defect in the body's steroidogenesis system and may be either partial or complete.

21:7 pill programme a method of administering oral contraceptives to women who take a pill containing the female sex hormones each day for 21 days, then stop for 7 days to permit menstruation to begin. 'Me woman begins the next cycle of 21 pills after 7 days regardless of when menstruation actually begins. The ritual helps the woman remember the routine because she always starts taking the contraceptive pills on the same day of the week. An alternative approach is to include 7 placebo pills to be taken between the 21-day contraceptive pills.

twins either of two general types of twins. fraternal, also called dizygotic or biovular; or identical, also called monozygotic or uniovular.

twixter an obsolete term for (a) a boyish girl or (b) a girlish boy.

two-backed boast, to do the an old literary term meaning to have face-to-face intercourse.

two-digit system a classification system for recording the number of times a woman has been pregnant and the number of viable off-spring. The system uses the symbols 0 and i separated by a solidus. Thus, a woman who is pregnant for the first time is recorded as 0/i; if the pregnancy ends with a viable infant, the record is changed to i/i. A second pregnancy is recorded as i/ii whether or not it is successfully carried to term. The system simply records parity/gravidity.

Type A and Type B the commonly identified psychological types of personality, with Type A representing the uptight, deadline-orientated individual and Type B the 'laid-back,' easy-going person. In tests of sexual behaviour by psychologists, it was found that Type A men could perform mathematical problems requiring concentration while listening to an erotic audiotape while Type B men were unable to concentrate on sexual and nonsexual events at the same time.

Tyson's glands the oil-secreting glands on the inner surfaces of the foreskin and the corona of the glans penis. The glandular secretion contributes to the formation of smegma; a lubricating substance.

Tzanck test a laboratory test for genital herpes, utilizing tissue scraped from a lesion. The tissue sample is stained with a dye that helps identify the herpes virus under a microscope.

U

umbilical cord the cord that connects the foetus with the placenta and provides a means for the flow of nutrients from the maternal blood supply to the foetus and for the removal of waste products from foetal metabolism. The umbilical cord is about 20 inches long and one inch thick and contains two arteries and one vein. The vein carries oxygenated blood to the foetus, and the arteries return the deoxygenated blood to the placenta. At birth, the umbilical cord is clamped or ligated and severed. The stump atrophies and falls off in about a week, leaving the navel, or belly button.

unconsummated marriage marriage in which the husband and wife have not had intercourse. In a study of 1,000 verified virgin wives, who had bee married between 1 and 21 years, it was found that the largest proportion cited fear of pain as a reason for avoiding intercourse (20 percent). The second most common reason (18 percent) was that sex was considered to be nasty or wicked. About 12 percent reported their husbands were impotent, 5 percent said that they were lesbians, and 9 percent expressed a general dislike of men or the penis or had a fear of semen. Nearly 14 percent indicated a lack of knowledge about sex anatomy, either misbelieving that the vagina was too small to accommodate an erect penis or claiming ignorance about the exact location of the female genitalia. Other reasons given by the women was a desire to be only a mother to the husband or that submitting to intercourse with a man would be interpreted as a loss of female equality or independence. When asked why they married a man in the first place, the virgin wives explained that they believed it was the proper thing to do, that they wanted to avoid being identified as an 'old maid', or that they did it for financial security. One quarter of the women admitted to participating in mutual masturbation with their husbands.

undersexed a colloquial term referring to a man or woman whose sex drive appears to be unusually weak. Though commonly attributed to an unspecified physical defect, the actual cause may be psychological—that is, inhibitions, inner conflicts, or distaste instilled during the individual's upbringing. In many cases, a person who is labelled under-sexed may be normally responsive if he or she finds the right partner. Technical terms are inhibited sexual desire, inhibited sexual excitement, inhibited female orgasm, and inhibited male orgasm.

undinism a rarely used term for a pathological interest in urine—as in urolagnia or urophilia.

unilateral sexual precocity a condition in which genitalia on one side of the body develop prematurely while the corresponding body parts on the opposite side develop at the normal rate. Thus, a girt may have an enlarged breast and mature labia with pubic hair on one side with no signs of precocity on the other. A corresponding type of condition is seen in cases of rudimentary testes.

uninhibited free from inhibitions, usually sexual or moral.

uniovular twins twins that develop from a single ovum. About 30 percent of all twins are uniovular although the manner in which they develop in the uterus can vary. A single fertilized ovum may separate into two blasto-meres resulting in two implantations with two placentas and two sets of membranes. The blastomeres may remain fused with two inner cell masses that implant with one chorion and one placenta but two separate amnions. Or, one blastomere with two inner cell masses may become implanted with a single placenta and shared amnion and chorion. Triplets or quadruplets also could develop from a single ovum, or from two, three, or four ova.

uniperous pertaining to a woman who has given birth only one time. The term has also been used to describe a delivery resulting in only one infant.

unisex an androgynous life-style in which men and women wear similar clothes, adopt similar hair styles, perform similar types of work, and share the same child rearing and other home responsibilities.

unisex toys that are neither male-nor female-oriented, such as building bricks, crayons or puzzles. They avoid the problem of sex-stereotyped toys for boys and girls.

unnatural acts a term sometimes applied by lawyers, legislators, or the public to sexual activities that they condemn, such as orogenital sex, anal intercourse, and homosexuality. The term is avoided by sexologists because it is moralistic rather than scientific and because it implies that nature has intentions that can be known and understood.

unpleasure a psychoanalytical term for the feelings of tension, discomfort and frustration that occur when instinctual impulses, such as hunger and sex, are denied gratification. The Gentian synonym, Unjust, is sometimes used by psychiatrists.

unsexed by failure a term introduced by Margaret Mead to describe a loss of sexual drive that often occurs in men who have failed to succeed at some endeavour. Being fired or retired from a job may have an effect of Psychological emasculation. The effect may be related to the so-called male menopause.

unwanted pregnancies a term referring to the number of undesired and usually unplanned children per couple. In the United States at Present the number of children unwanted by at least one parent has been conservatively estimated at over one million per year, and the number born to poor parents has been estimated at double the number born to the more affluent.

unwed chic a colloquial term referring to a young unmarried mother who is economically and socially able to become pregnant and support a child without the benefit of legal ties to a husband.

unwed father the father of the child of an unmarried mother.

upper lip according to Tantric and Japanese doctrines, one of the most erogenous areas of the female body. Hindu treatises claim there is a 'secret nerve' connecting the clitoris to the upper lip, and that a woman can enhance the pleasures of lovemaking both for herself and her partner by stimulating this nerve through deep alternate-nostril breathing.

uranism an obsolete term for homosexuality, especially in the male, coined by Karl Heinrich Ulrichs in 1862, and derived from Aphrodite Urania, the goddess of heavenly love in Greek mythology. Two other term were derived from the same source: urning applied to a male homosexual who plays the female role with other males; and urninde applied to a female homosexual who plays the passive role with other females.

urosplasmsa urealyticum a species of very small bacteria that cause genital-tract infections in both men and women.

urethra the channel through which untie passes from the urinary bladder. The female urethra is relatively short, a little more than one inch in length. It exists in front of the vaginal onfice. The male urethra is about 8 inches long and is divided into dim segments. The first, the prostatic portion, runs more or less vertically for if bit more than one inch through the prostate gland. In the prostatic segment the male urethra is perforated by openings from the prostate-gland ducts and the seminal vesicles. Next is a short membranous portion of less than one inch between the prostate and the bulb of the penis, In the membranous portion the urethra passes through the urethral sphincter. The third segment is within the corpus spongiosurn of the penile shaft. Congenital defects found occasionally in the corpus spongiosumportion are clefts that direct the urine from the undersurface or upper surface of the shaft of the penis.

urethral abscess an abscess in the submucosal layer

of tissue lining the urethra as a result of an infection such as gonorrhoea. In the male urethra, an abscess frequently develops in the midportion of the penis producing a visible swelling.

urethral character a Freudian term for a personality pattern characterized by a long history of bed-wetting and a set of traits stemming from feelings of shame associated with incontinence as well as the fear of urethral eroticism—namely, overambitiousness and boastfulness. These character traits are interpreted as an attempt to reestablish the bed wetter's self-esteem.

urethral chill a chill experienced by persons as a result of the entry of bacterial or other foreign products into the circulation via the corpus spongiosum. The urethral chill is often associated with the insertion of catheters of instruments into the penile urethra. It also may be a sign of damage to the lining of the urethra, permitting urine, pus, or other substances to infiltrate the surrounding tissues.

urethral eroticism a psychoanalytical term for sexual Pleasure accompanying urination. A person who remains fixated at the urethral stage of psychosexual development may develop fantasies or wishes concerning urinating on other people, or being urinated on.

urethral groove the lower surface of the embryonic penis which normally closes to form the Penile segment of the urethra. If the groove fails to close, it results in the congenital defect of hypospadias.

urethral insertion introduction of an object such as a pin or match stick into the urethra during masturbation or as a form of masturbation. The practice is occasionally found among boys and girls but is highly dangerous. Medical assistance and possibly surgery may be required.

urethral stage the phase of psychosexual development that occurs between the anal and phallic stages, when the urethra becomes the prime erogenous zone and sexual pleasure is derived from urinating. At this stage the child frequently comes into conflict with the parents over bladder training, and feels humiliated when he or she cannot exercise control or wets the bed.

urethritis an inflammation of the urethra, usually producing pus cells that indicate infection by bacteria Chlamydia trachomatis, fungi viruses chemicals, protozoa or objects inserted in the urethra for purposes of masturbation.

urethrovaginal meatus an anomaly associated with some cases of hermaphroditism in which a well-developed clitoris resembles a penis with hypospadias. The opening of the urethra is at the base of the clitoris. Because of the similarity between the labia and a scrotum, some females born with this congenital defect have been judged hypospadiac males at birth.

urinary responses the reactions of the urinary system to sexual excitement. In women, the urethra may undergo a few feeble contractions during orgasm. The urethra of the male is an important part of the penis and is quite sensitive to sexual activity. The urge to urinate after orgasm is common and may be aggravated in some cases because of irritation to the bladder during the body pressures and frictions of sexual intercourse.

urinary-tract infection any infection involving all or a portion of the urinary system, from the kidneys to the urethra. Urinary-tract infections are generally bacterial in origin and in adults are likely to enter the body through the urethra. In children, the infection usually enters the urinary tract from the blood vessels or lymphatic system. Kinds of urinary-tract infections include miliary tuberculosis, vesical mycoses, gonorrhoea, group A streptococcus, Escherichia coli, staphylococcus, Candida, and Chlamydia. Urinary-tract infections are relatively rare in men, except for those with spinal-cord injuries, but women are frequently at risk from such infections.

urination and sex a term referring to the observing of urination (in male or female)—an early, and usually surreptitious, expression of interest in sex and the sex organs. In some instances this interest may develop into a paraphilia known as urolagnia, characterized by a morbid preoccupation with urine and urination, especially as a means of sexual excitement.

urinism a sexual practice in which urine or urination plays a part in the sexual act, as in urinating on one's partner, watching the partner urinate during foreplay, urinating during intercourse (women only), or smelling urine on the body or clothes of the partner.

urninde and urning two terms for types of homosexuality derived from the name of the goddess Aphrodite Urania.

urogeital chamber a structure in the embryonic stage of human development in which the primitive genital and urinary organs share a common opening.

urogenital diaphragm a layer of tissue that forms a floor at the bottom of the pelvic cavity within a triangular area consisting of the lower edges of the pelvic bones, from the ischial tuberosities on either side of the anus to the symphysis pubis beneath the bulb of the penis. The deep transverse perineal muscle lies between layers of connective tissue of the diaphragm.

urogenital-floor muscles a group of five muscles in the male that participate in the clonic spasms of semen ejaculation. They include the bulbocavernosus, the sphincter urethrae, erector penis, transversus perineiprofundus, and transversus perinei superficialis. A similar group of urogenital muscles are found in the female, where the bulbocavernosus is known as the sphincter vaginae, and the ischiocavernosus is identified as the erector clitoridis.

urogenital sinus a primordial structure in the embryo that later develops into either male or female genital features. In the male, the urogenital sinus evolves into the prostate, the prostatic utricle, and the Cowper glands. In the female, the same structure develops into the lower vagina, the paraurethral glands, and Bartholin's glands.

urolagnia a sexual deviation, or paraphilia, characterized by a morbid attraction for the urine or the urinary processes of the sex partner or other individuals. Sexual stimulation may be experienced by watching the partner urinate, by sniffing garments smelling of urine during intercourse or masturbation, by drinking the partner's urine, or by yielding to one's desire or the partner's desire to be urinated upon.

urophilia a psychosexual disorder consisting of an

obsessive interest in urine and urination as a source of sexual excitement.

uterine angle the portion of the uterus surrounding the openings of the fallopian tubes.

uterine axis a hypothetical line running through the longest diameter of the uterus.

uterine cavity the hollow portion of the uterus, including the cervical canal.

uterine displacement a shift from the normal position of the uterus in the pelvic cavity, usually because of failure of the ligaments to maintain the womb in the normal position-at right angles to the vagina and horizontal when the woman is standing. Displacement of the uterus can result in painful menstruation, pelvic congestion, backache, and discomfort during coitus.

uterine-hernia syndrome a condition in which a person with normal male sexual characteristics, including the ability to produce sperm, also possesses a uterus and fallopian tubes. In most cases, the condition is not discovered until surgery is required or an inguinal hernia or other disorder develops that involves an incision into the pelvic area.

uterine sinus a blood-filled space in the pregnant uterus.

uteroplacental insufficiency any disorder of the placenta that renders it incapable of supporting foetal life. Causes may be hormonal insufficiency, an infection, or an interference with the blood supply. Placentitis may result from a bacterial, viral, rickettsial, or protozoal infection. Deposition of fibrin around the villi can inactivate the villi, thereby eliminating the maternal blood circulation.

uterosacral ligaments strong cords of fibrous tissue that follow a curved course from the uterine cervix to the sacrum, at the lower end of the spinal column, along the wall of the pelvis. The ligaments help support the uterus.

uterovaginal canal a structure in the embryo that evolves into vagina, uterus, and fallopian tubes of the female. In the male, the canal atrophies but leaves vestiges of tissue on the testis and the prostate.

uterus a hollow muscular organ with thick walls located in the pelvic region of the female; the structure in which a fertilized ovum is nurtured into a viable individual. In a nonpregnant woman, the uterus is a small pear-shaped organ, about 3 inches in length, which protrudes at the cervical end into the vault of the vagina. Two fallopian tubes, or oviducts, are attached to the uterus at both sides less than 1 inch from the top, or fundus. The portion below the level of the tubes is the body of the uterus, except for the cervix, and round neck of the womb that extends into the vagina. The proportions of corpus, or body, and cervix, change between childhood and motherhood. In a female child, the cervix represents about two thirds of the uterus. In a nonpregnant young woman, the uterus is divided so that about half is body and half cervix. After pregnancy, one third is cervix and two thirds are uterine body.

uterus bicornis unicollis a congenital anomaly in which a single uterine cervix leads into two adjacent uterine organs. Each side of the duplex uterus is attached to one of the fallopian tubes.

uterus didelphys a congenital anomaly in which two normal uteruses develop. Each uterus receives a fallopian tube from its side of the pelvic cavity. And each fallopian tube is attached to one ovary. The separate uteruses function independently and each is capable of supporting a pregnancy.

uterus duplex bicornis a congenital anomaly in which a pair of uteruses develop side by side, each attached to one of the fallopian tubes. However, unlike the uterus didelphys, which consists of completely separate reproductive organs, the uterus duplex bicornis consists of a uterus on either side of a thick wall of myometrium that is shared by both uteruses.

uterus masculinus an alternative term for the male prostatic utricle, which is believed to be homologous with the uterus and vagina of the female.

uterus septus a pair of fused uteruses with a single cervix but divided by a wall of muscle tissue. The wall, or septum, extends to the cervical opening.

uterus subseptus a uterus that is parfly divided down the centre by a wall of tissue. Unlike the septum in the uterus septus, the uterus subseptus contains a dividing wall that extends from the fundus to a point about halfway through the uterine cavity.

uterus unicornis a congenital anomaly in which a normal functioning uterus develops with only one fallopian tube attached.

V

vagina a musculomembranous tube that is a passageway between the uterine cervix and the vaginal orifice. It develops from early in the foetal period through puberty into a thin walled tube about four inches in length and less than two inches in width, with the cervix extending nearly one inch into the vault of the tube. The vagina is located anatomically between the bladder and the rectum and is supported by ligaments and muscles of the pelvic floor. Its walls are formed by an internal mucous membrane lining and a muscular coat, with a layer of erectile tissue between them. The mucous membrane lining is continuous with that of the uterus. It is not a smooth surface but rather one that is marked by ridges and furrows. The ridges are sometimes identified as the columns of the vagina, and also as rugae. It contains a number of mucous crypts, but there are no glands within the vagina. The muscular coat consists of an external layer of longitudinal fibres that are continuous with the muscles of the uterus and an internal layer of circular fibres. The erectile tissue is provided by fibres of the bulbocavernosus muscle. The main functions of the vagina are to provide a passageway for spermatozoa from the penis, an outlet for the menstrual flow from the uterus, and a birth canal for the foetus at term. The vaginal lining responds to stimulation by the female sex hormones oestrogen and progesterone. As a result, there is some proliferation and exfoliation of the mucosa during the menstrual cycle. Because the mucosal lining of the uterus is continuous with that of the vagina, a sample of vaginal tissue is regarded as a reliable source for information about the condition of the endometriurn of the uterus, particularly with regard for effects of the sex hormones. A scraping of vaginal mucus is often included with the cervical scraping when a sample of tissue is required for a smear test for cancer. But the vagina itself is rarely a source of cancer. It is, however, a potential source for parasitic and pathogenic organisms, particularly those associated with sexually transmissible diseases.

vagina dentata in psychoanalysis, the fantasy—more unconscious than conscious—that the vagina contains teeth that can castrate the male partner. In males, this fantasy is believed to be based on castration anxiety; and in females it is believed to stem from penis envy and a desire to castrate the male as an act of revenge.

vaginal adhesions a condition associated with the postmenopausal senile vagina in which firm fibrous growths descend from the upper vagina, forming attachments across the lumen (opening) of the vagina, and eventually obscuring and obstructing the vaginal canal.

vaginal ballottement a method of examining the condition of a pregnancy by producing a movement in the amniotic fluid through the walls of the vagina. By initiating movement of the amniotic fluid, the examiner can obtain information about the foetus whose movements respond to the fluid activity because the foetus is of about the same specific gravity as the fluid in which it is suspended.

vaginal balls a sexual device for women that consists of two weighted plastic spheres, each about one inch in diameter attached to a cord joined to a waist belt. The balls are inserted in the vagina (and in some cases in the rectum) and the woman derives sexual pleasure, usually to the point of repeated orgasm, by walking back and forth or rocking in a chair. The device is said to have originated in Japan.

vaginal bulb the embryonic tissue mass that forms at the end of the uterovaginal canal. It is usually visible in the foetus during the seventh week of gestation.

vaginal canal the tubular structure formed by the walls of the vagina.

vaginal columns the transverse ridges of mucosal tissue on the walls of the vagina.

vaginal creams medicated ointments containing female hormones that may be applied to the vagina to act as a lubricant thereby reducing the discomfort of dyspareunia.

vaginal discharge the flow of any substance from the vagina, usually excluding the natural menstrual flow. The term is commonly applied to irritating discharges that are associated with infections. Leukorrhoea, a whitish discharge consisting of and discarded cells of the vaginal lining, may be normal if it occurs during pregnancy, just before menstruation, or during ovulation, unless the flow is copious. Abnormal vaginal discharges are associated with trichomonas vaginitis, a leukorrhoea that is irritating and causes swelling of the, vaginal tissues and painful intercourse; monilial vaginitis, which also is irritating and a cause of painful intercourse, and gonorrhoea. Lochia is a normal vaginal discharge that occurs after child delivery and may persist for several weeks, changing in colour from red to brown to a yellowish white during the first two weeks after labour.

vaginal envy a form of envy experienced particularly by male transsexuals who not only have a persistent desire to be rid of their own genitals, but also to possess the sexual organs of the female including the vagina.

vaginal epithelioma a type of vaginal cancer that begins as a small ulceration or pimply growth on the wall of the vagina. Untreated, it tends to spread wildly through the vaginal walls to invade other organs and tissues of the pelvic cavity.

vaginal examination the study of the vagina for the possible presence of anomalies, infections or other diseases, and to determine its role as a possible infertility factor. A routine digital examination of the vagina often is not feasible before puberty because of the presence of the hymen. A long, thin, lighted vaginoscope may be inserted through a perforation in the hymen, allowing a superficial prepubertal examination. At puberty, the hymenal opening is usually larger and the vaginal wall more distensible so that a finger or thin vaginal speculum can be inserted. After puberty, the vaginal examination is performed as part of a complete pelvic examination for evidence of infections, tumours, vaginismus, infertility, and dyspareunia. The presence of an infection, such as *Trichomonas vaginalis* can cause the vagina to be too alkaline for the male spermatozoa, to survive. The study of the vaginal canal may indicate whether a healthy male ejaculate would likely be deposited in the area of the vagina next to the opening of the cervix. A narrow vagina, for example, could prevent the penis from reaching the optimum portion of the vagina and that problem could be compounded if the male happened to suffer from erectile dysfunction or premature ejaculation. A malpositioned uterus or a cervix that is too high in the vagina could also be obstacles to fertilization of an ovum and would be detected by a vaginal examination. The examination might reveal the presence of a polyp or other lesion that could obstruct the passage of spermatozoa. Other observable factors may be signs of an infection and excessive mucus production, which can be a cause of infertility. A cervix that is tapered with a tiny opening is a sign of an undeveloped uterus and would be noticed during a vaginal examination.

vaginal father a psychoanalytical term for a male who dreams or fantasizes that he has a vagina. This notion is believed to stem from an unconscious identification with the man's own mother, and is associated with motherly, unaggressive behaviour, intense rivalry with women, and a predilection for homemaking and child rearing in marriage.

vaginal fistula an abnormal passageway that develops through the vaginal wall so that it connects directly with neighbouring organs, such as the rectum or the urinary bladder. The fistula may be congenital or may result from a tumour or injury related to surgery or child delivery.

vaginal fluid another term for vaginal lubrication.

vaginal hypoaesthesia a form of partial frigidity in which sexual sensitivity is limited to the clitoral area.

vaginal insertions the insertion of fingers or objects into the vagina during masturbation. Kinsey found that one in five women reported such insertions—most frequently the fingers, but also easily available objects such as pencils, bananas, or candles and in some cases artificial penises.

Vagina Littlefinger a male homosexual slang term for a snob.

vaginal lubrication secretion of lubricating fluid by the vaginal walls and Bartholin's glands situated on each side of the vaginal orifice. The process is also known as 'sweating' and occurs during the excitement stage of the sexual-response cycle making coitus easier to perform.

vaginal melanoma a particularly dangerous type of pigmented tumour that may develop in the vagina. It is a lethal type of cancer and one that is always secondary to a melanoma that first appeared in some other body area. But it is distinctively out of place in the vagina, because of its dark mole like appearance, and easy to detect in its earliest stages.

vagina loquens in ancient folklore, a vagina that is forced, through a charm, to speak and thus reveal its lack of chastity (telling all about her lovers).

vaginal orgasm a climax reportedly experienced by the woman through stimulation of the vagina alone, without any clitoral stimulation. According to Freud, only a vaginal orgasm, as distinguished from a clitoral orgasm, can be called 'mature' and 'real'. This view, as well as the view that there is a separate and distinct vaginal orgasm, has been challenged by Kinsey and by Masters and Johnson.

vaginal plethysmograph a device that measures the sexual arousal in a female by data obtained from changes in blood flow and erectile-tissue changes in the vagina.

vaginal sarcoma a type of cancer of the vagina that may develop in the muscle or subcutaneous layers of the posterior vaginal wall. It grows so rapidly that portions may slough off because of a lack of blood supply. It may spread by metastasis to the lungs or other parts of the body.

vaginal secretion a clear fluid secreted by the vaginal barrel during sexual excitement. Contractions of the vaginal muscles often bring the walls together so sharply that the secretions spurt out of the vagina. This is the source of the mistaken notion that women ejaculate like men.

vaginal suppository a cone-shaped medical preparation that is melted by the body heat when introduced into the vagina before intercourse. Though suppositories of this kind provide a barrier against sperm, and contain a spermicide, they are not regarded as an effective contraceptive.

vaginismus a painful spasm of the vagina, usually of emotional origin. It can interfere with satisfactory intercourse or with a routine pelvic examination. It involves an intense contraction of the muscle fibres surrounding the vagina.

vaginitis any inflammation of the lining of the

vagina resulting from atrophy, infection, physical injury. Infectious agents may include *Haemophilus vaginalis,* primarily a parasitic organism but one that produces a malodorous leukorrhoea. Amoebic vaginitis is caused by *Entamoeba histolytica* an organism that causes ulcerations of the vagina and cervix. Vaginitis may result from Listeria monocytogenes, which is harboured in the vagina of a significant percentage of women, particularly in the summer and autumn. Simple vaginitis may be caused by Escherichia coli one of several disease agents that alter the acidity of the lining of the vagina to produce symptoms of burning, itching, and swelling, with pain or urination. Monlial vaginitis is associated Candida albicans, a fungal infection that causes a thick discharge that produces itching and irritation and usually results in dyspareunia, or pain during intercourse. Trichomonas vaginitis is a protozoan that also produces a discharge and irritation and causes dyspareunia. Some other forms of vaginitis are caused by pediculosis pubis, the crab louse, and by the we of clothing and cosmetics, mainly deodorants, that create an allergic reaction. Adhesive vaginitis is caused by walls of the vagina that stick together. Atrophic vaginitis is an effect of the menopause when decreased oestrogen levels result in a thinning and increased sensitivity of the mucosal lining.

valerian a herb generally associated with sexual stimulation, also known as 'drunken sailor'. This alleged aphrodisiac was administered by witches; and as 'cetwale' in Chaucer's *Canterbury, Tales* it was a herb to be added to ale to cause lovelonging. The herb, whose name is derived from the *Latin valere,* meaning 'to be well,' was known to ancient

Greeks and Romans and was used as a source of medicine, by monks in the Middle Ages.

vampirism belief in the existence of preter-natural beings who arise from the ground and fly around like bats, sucking the blood of sleeping persons. Drawing, and drinking, blood is believed to be a means of achieving sexual gratification. Some writers regard the practice of biting the partner during sexual activity as a form of vampirism.

vanilla a plant that is related botanically to the orchid and which, for that reason, has been thought to be an aphrodisiac. Next to celery soup and chocolate, Madame Pompadour recommended the use of vanilla, in fact, she flavoured her chocolate with vanilla extract.

variant sexual behaviour a recently coined expression used by sexologists and sex educators for sexual behaviour that is not engaged in by most People. It is a purely descriptive term, not implying right or wrong or abnormality, in contradistinction to older terms like deviant, perverted, or unnatural.

varicocale a large varicose vein in the scrotum that is associated with as many as 40 percent of cases of male infertility. Surgical correction of a varicocele reportedly increases the sperm count in half the cases.

varicose vulva an abnormal condition in which the vulva becomes swollen because of an impeded return flow of blood. The condition stems from or is aggravated by repeated pregnancies that cause increased pressure of blood vessels in the lower pelvis. Varicose veins of the vulva may appear only when a woman is standing and subside when she lies on her back. There are hazards of a rupture of one of the varicose veins or formation of blood clots in the vulva.

vasa efferentia an alternative term for the efferent ducts of the rete testis, through which the mature spermatozoa move into the epididymis.

vas deferens an alternative term for ductus deferens, a long muscular tube that carries spermatozoa from the epididymis to the urethral portion of the prostate gland.

vasectomy a male sterilization procedure in which the vas deferens (ductus, deferens) is divided within the male scrotum. The procedure takes less than 15 minutes in most cases and requires a local anaesthetic. The genital area is cleaned and shaved to reduce the risk of infection. An anaesthetic is injected into the scrotal skin and again into each vas deferens after it has been located within the scrotal tissues. The vas may be simply severed or a small section may be excised. Some doctors irrigate the opened vas to decrease the postoperative sperm count using xylocaine or another substance, such as a salt solution. Vasectomized men treated with xylocaine irrigation of the vas are azoospermic within 6 weeks after the procedure, whereas untreated vasectomized men required up to 10 weeks to produce semen free of motile spermatozoa. After irrigation, the vas ends may be sealed by one of three standard methods: by ligation, or tying the open ends with sutures; by coagulation with electricity or heat; or by applying tantalum clips. Some doctors apply clips without severing the vas while others sever the vas, irrigate, and cauterize before applying clips. The patient is advised to rest for a couple of hours after a vasectomy and to avoid strenuous physical work or exercise for several days. For postoperative discomfort, doctors may recommend wearing a scrotal support for a week and taking aspirin or other easily available analgesics. Because some doctors perform a vasectomy with a single incision into the scrotum whereas others make a separate incision for each vas deferens, plus other individual fact, the rate of healing varies somewhat. However, the man is allowed to resume intercourse as soon as he feels comfortable in that activity. Unlike female sterilization, a vasectomy does not have immediate results. Spermatozoa stored anywhere along the reproductive tract beyond the point of the vas division car result in a pregnancy. Pregnancies have occurred more than 1 month after a vasectomy, and whereas 95 percent of vasectomized men are azoospermic after 10 weeks, the other 5 percent may still ejaculate spermatozoa. In the United States, doctors performing vasectomies frequently request a sperm Sample 7 or 8 weeks after the operation for examination. In other countries, men are advised to continue using other forms of contraception for a period of 3 months after the vasectomy. A vasectomy is usually permanent, but some surgeons report a 50 percent success in reversing the procedure.

vasocongestion the engorgement of spongy erectile tissues of the penis and clitoris with blood. By automatic manipulation of the blood flow by spinal nerve tracts, arteries allow blood to move into the spongy tissues faster than it is allowed to drain through the veins, as occurs when the penis is flaccid. Valves in the veins also retard the return flow of blood, which is required to produce turgidity in the erectile tissues.

vasconstrictor centres a part of the sympathetic

nervous system, located in the lumbar area of the spinal cord. The vasoconstrictor centres prevent blood entering the penis or clitoris from leaving during the erection phase of sexual stimulation. By allowing an inflow of blood while preventing an outflow, the penis can remain turgid and still during intercourse.

vasodilator centres a part of the parasympathetic nervous system, located in the sacral nerve areas of the spinal cord, that controls the flow of blood into the penis or clitoris during the erection phase of sexual arousal.

Vatican roulette a colloquial term for the rhythm method of birth control, which depends upon avoiding intercourse around the time of ovulation. It is the only method permitted by the Roman Catholic Church.

VD a common abbreviation for venereal disease.

vegetarian a slang term for a person who does not like to perform fellatio or cunnilingus.

veil wearing the practice of covering the face of women with a cloth or veil as a sexual shield and a means of keeping them in seclusion and subservience. Once common in Muslim societies, the veil is slowly disappearing, although it has been retained or reintroduced by fundamentalists, as in Iran. In Chad, some non-Muslim women wear an elaborate beaded veil, but wear nothing else; and among the Tuareg of the Sahara only the men wear veils.

vena cave syndrome a condition that occurs in a normal pregnant woman during the third trimester when she lies on her back so that the bulk of the uterus passes on the inferior vena cava, the major vein of the lower part of the body. The inferior vena cava is compressed against the spinal column, reducing the return flow of blood to the mother's heart. This condition, in turn, results in falling blood pressure so that less blood can reach the placenta, causing foetal distress.

venereal disease (VD) a popular term for sexually transmitted disease.

venereal-disease phobia a more common term for cypridophobia.

venery an obsolete term for indulgence in sexual intercourse.

venetian blinds a homosexual slang term for foreskin.

ventral-dorsal a coital position in which intercourse is performed with one partner facing the back of the other.

ventral-ventral an alternative term for the coital position in which the partners face each other.

Venus the ancient Roman goddess associated with love. Born of the sea, she has often been linked with the belief that fish are a powerful erotic aid. So deeply rooted is the association between Venus and the aphrodisiac value of seafood that the eating of seafood was prohibited by religious leaders on several occasions in history, including the beginning of the Christian era, when church officials tried to eradicate ties with the Roman past.

Venus' highway an older euphemism for vagina, especially a prostitutes.

verbal masochism a form of masochism in which a person seeks or actually achieves sexual excitement by imagining he or she is a target for insults and other forms of verbal abuse. Some mental patients dwell on the same masochistic fantasies and dialogues for years because they find them sexually exciting.

version a change in the lie, or position, of he foetus in the uterus. The change is usually manipulated by the physician to make the delivery easier. Three basic types of version are cephalic, podalic, or combined. A cephalic version is one in which the foetus in a breech or transverse position across the cervical outlet is manoeuvred so that the feet and buttocks are at the top of the uterus and the cephalic, or head, portion is pointed downwards into the birth canal. A cephalic version is manipulated externally by gently pushing he buttocks upwards and the head downwards through palpation of the foetal body through the mother's abdominal wall. The manoeuvre reduces the risk of a foetal loss from 15 to 3 percent. The podalic version accomplishes a similar objective, but the manipulation is performed internally, usually by reaching into the uterus and grasping the feet of the foetus. The combined version, as the name suggests, involves both external and internal manipulation of the foetus within the uterus. Because of improved techniques and safety, a caesarean section is preferred by most modern obstetricians to the internal or combined forms of version.

verumontanitis an inflammation of the verumontanum, located on the floor of the urethra near the prostate. Among causes are excessive sexual activity prostatitis, and seminal vesculitis. If the swelling blocks the ejaculatory ducts, the man may experience pain radiation to the lower back, perineum, and scrotum. Urinary frequency and premature ejaculation are sometimes caused by verumontanitis.

verumontanum an elevated portion of the back wall of the prostatic urethra, at the point where the ejaculatory ducts and the prostatic utricle open into the urethra.

vestibular glands a pair of small glands located on both sides of the vaginal orifice or opening. The term may also be applied to numerous snail mucous glands that open into the vestibule of the vagina.

vestibule a space leading to an entrance, such as the vestibule of the vagina, the space enclosed by the labia minora.

vestibulovaginal bulb a long mass of erectile tissue an both sides of the orifice of the vagina. Also called bulb of the vestibule.

vibrator a motor-driven plastic cylinder used mainly to transmit vibrations to the clitoris directly or through the hand. A penis-shaped vibrator is used- and often recommended by sex therapists—to produce an orgasm in women (also men) who have not had this experience, or who are having difficulty reaching orgasm through other forms of stimulation. Some women, however, find the instrument too mechanical for their taste. A smaller version is sometimes used for anal stimulation.

vicarious menstruation an unusual condition in which bleeding from the nose or other parts of the body, such as the eyes, occurs during the menstrual flow, presumably caused either by psychological factor by a vasospasm that results in a sudden decrease in the size of the blood vessels of the endometriurn.

vice a term referring to any practice that a particular society considers to be depraved or immoral—often used with another word, as in 'secret vice', which was probably the most common 19th century euphemism for masturbation.

Victorianism stereotyped attitudes prevalent in Western nations during the age of Queen Victoria, who reigned from 1837 to 1901. The term includes the notion that sex, itself is ugly or 'beastly,' that only loose women enjoy it, that nice, women must avoid, getting sexually excited, that they tolerate sexual relations only as a necessary evil and a duty to their husbands and that sex is something one doesn't talk about in polite society or even behind closed doors. As a result prudery were triumphant, books and play were censored, children were kept complete ignorance of sexual matters, lovers were chaperoned, and women wore bathing attire that covered their legs down to their ankles.

viraginity a term pertaining to a woman with the physical characteristics of a man.

virgin an individual, male or female, who has not engaged in sexual intercourse. Virginity, or premarital chastity, is regarded as essential in Islamic societies, and is, greatly emphasized by many parents arid some young people in our own culture. Virginity was regarded as a sacred state by the Romans, who appointed the vestal virgins to deal with the gods. On the other hand, many societies do not consider virginity to be important, and some even require women to prove their fertility by having a child before marriage.

Virgin is also a slang term for a couple or a partner not experienced in group sex or 'swinging'—that is, greenhorns in this practice.

virginal anxiety a state of apprehension experienced by a girl or woman during her first sexual encounter.

virgin birth the concept of human pregnancy and subsequent birth without a union of ovum and sperm after intercourse. The belief in the virgin birth of Jesus appears to be a reflection of the view that equates virginity with purity. The nearest thing to virgin birth is impregnation without penile penetration: This has been known to occur when the man ejaculates near or on a virgin's vulva during sex play, or if he gets semen on his hands and then brings his fingers into contact with her vagina.

virginity taboo a social prohibition against defloration of the woman before marriage. This taboo is by no means universal; for example, an anthropological study of 141 non-Western societies conducted by Broude and Greene has shown that these societies were about evenly divided on the question of premarital virginity. In Western societies a woman was expected to be virginal before marriage until the 1950s. Since that the number of nonvirgins at marriage has rapidly risen and appears to be well over 50 percent at present.

virilescence the gradual appearance of male characteristics, such as facial hair and a deeper voice, in a woman, particularly after menopause.

virilism a condition of women possessing masculine characteristics, such as an enlarged clitoris, deep voice, male hairline, and general masculine body shape, in addition to hirsutism.

virility the capacity for sexual functioning in the male; male potency.

virtue admirable quality or moral excellence. Literally, the term means manliness, a male's strength or merit, from Latin vir, meaning 'adult male'. Ironically, however, the term virtue has come to refer primarily to women—perhaps as an expression of male chauvinist' expectations.

vital strength a term referring to the energy that some men mistakenly believe is discharged along with semen during ejaculation. It is pan of a myth that a man is born with a fixed number of possible orgasms in to reproductive system and that he become increasingly debilitated in later life because of this loss of 'vital strength'.

voice change the deepening and maturing of the male voice and, less obviously, the female voice during puberty. In boys this occurs during the rapid growth spurt of the whole body; more specifically, the enlargement of the voice box is the result of an increase in male hormone secretion from the testicles. The change usually becomes noticeable several months after the first ejaculation. In the case of castration, the male hormones cease to be produced, and voice pitch increases. On the other hand, neoplasms of the ovaries may result in a masculine lowering of the female voice.

voluptas sexualis a Latin term meaning sexual pleasure, found mainly in 19th century literature.

von Fernwald's sign a pregnancy sign noted during the eighth week of gestation by a bulge on a side of the top of the uterus, the site of implantation of the embryo.

Voronoff, Serge one of several experimenters in rejuvenation techniques based on the transplantation of animal gonads into humans.

Voronoff, a Russian doctor, worked in the 1920's at implanting ape testicles in humans to increase or restore male potency— but was not successful.

voyeurism a sexual disorder in which an individual, usually a male—a voyeur—derives sexual satisfaction from secretly observing people in the nude, or in the act of undressing or engaging in sexual activity. If this is the preferred or exclusive method of achieving sexual excitement, it is classified as a paraphilia.

voyuse a female voyeur.

vulcanization the discovery in 1843 of a method for processing flexible rubber products. The new process made possible the large-scale manufacture of rubber condoms, replacing the traditional types made of linen, animal intestines, or other substances. The first rubber condoms were moulded from crepe rubber and carried a seam lengthwise. It was not until the end of the 19th century that seamless rubber condoms became available.

vulva the external female vagina, and Bartholin's glands. In addition sex organs, or genitalia, comprising the mons veneris, the labia majora and minora, the clitoris, the vestibule or opening of vagina and Bartholin's glands.

W

wand a male homosexual slang term for penis.

Wands Wandwaver a male homosexual slang term for someone who brags about his penis size or performance.

wandering uterus a term applied to variations in the position of the uterus, which is normally at right angles to the axis of the vagina. A shift to an unusual position may cause painful menstruation, backaches, and pelvic congestion, and may also make intercourse uncomfortable.

Wandervogel movement an early 20th century youth movement in Germany in which nudism was practised. Wandervogel groups, which resembled the Scouts, denied charges of licentiousness and homosexuality that were levelled at them.

wank a slang term meaning to masturbate or masturbation In addition to being a masturbator, a wanker is a dilettante and also more generally a useless incompetent person.

werfarin a coumarin-type of anticoagulant drug sometimes prescribed for the treatment of coronary thrombosis and related cardiovascular disorders. Its use is contraindicated in women who are pregnant or capable of becoming pregnant because of its teratogenic effects on the offspring, including blindness and mental deficiency.

watering-can perineum medical jargon for a urethral abnormality in which strictures of the urinary pathway have led to multiple fistulas that permit the urine to spray from several openings at once.

waters a euphemism for the amniotic fluid within a pregnant woman's uterus, used particularly in the phrase 'breaking of the waters' referring to the rupture of the membranes containing this fluid.

water sports a slang term referring to sexual fascination with urine and urination, often abbreviated as w/s.

W chromosome a female sex hormone of certain animals, particularly birds, fishes, and insects. Unlike human females who possess duplicate (XX) sex chromosomes, females with a W chromosome received only one sex chromosome which must be paired with a Z chromosome, the male sex chromosome of the species. The WZ letters were assigned to such animals to distinguish their sex chromosomes from the XY or XX sets of human sex chromosomes.

wedding depression feelings of dejection and loss of initiative experienced by prospective brides and bridegrooms while plans for the wedding are in progress. This condition is presumably caused by such factors as apprehensiveness about taking on new responsibilities and the prospect of leaving the security of the family home. The depressed mood usually clears up spontaneously, but if it persists and is accompanied by insomnia and weight loss, professional assistance will generally be required.

wedding night the night after the marriage ceremony, when the couple are 'alone at last.' Traditionally, this night marks the beginning of sexual adjustment between the bride and groom. If one or both are virginal, the wedding night may be disappointing or stressful, particularly if they expect to 'reach the stars' immediately. But if they are mature enough to recognize that the sexual relationship takes time to develop—and is intertwined with their total relationship—they will be as realistic as they are romantic. Even those who have already experienced sexual relations with each other, or with other persons, usually find that marriage brings with it new circumstances and new responsibilities from the wedding night on.

wedding tackle a humorous euphemism for the male genitals.

wee-wee a euphemism meaning urine or to urinate, by or to children. The shorter wee is used similarly.

Weinberg and Williams Survey a large scale study of male homosexuals conducted in the 1970s in the United States and Europe under the sponsorship of the Kinsey Institute. Male homosexuals in the United States were contacted through mailing lists of the Mattachine Societies of New York and San Francisco. European homosexuals were interviewed in Amsterdam and Copenhagen. Data were obtained from more than 1,000 male homosexuals.

well hung an appreciative slang term describing a man with large genitalia or a woman with large breasts.

wet day a day in the menstrual cycle when cervical mucus secretion has increased and has become less clear and less sticky than in previous days that were still considered relatively free of risk of pregnancy. For women who use the ovulation method of family planning, wet days may indicate that ovulation is about to occur and intercourse should be avoided unless the woman wants to become pregnant.

wet dream an alternative term for nocturnal emission, a seminal discharge that accompanies an erotic dream by a male.

wet nurse a woman who breast-feeds an infant that is not her own child.

wet kiss a sexually stimulating kiss performed with wet lips and wet tongues.

wham-bang-thankyou-ma'am a derogatory term for the male attitude towards sexual intercourse as something to be indulged in for speedy and selfish gratification, with no thought for affection towards or the feelings of one's partner.

whipping lashing another person (or being lashed) with a whip, belt, thong, or other object, especially for the purpose of sexual arousal and gratification, as in dippoldism, flagellation, flagellantism, and flogging.

white-oak leaves leaves with alleged erotic properties. Women in 18th century England were advised to place two white-oak leaves on their pillow on the evening of Saint Valentine's Day. The leaves presumably would help the woman see her lover in her dreams that night.

white slave a young woman who has been forced into prostitution. The term is apparently derived from a 19th century drama entitled The White Slave, a story about a woman who was kidnapped and forced to be a prostitute. Because the story was set in the 1850s, it was necessary to distinguish white slavery, an illegal practice then, from black slavery.

white tunic an alternative term for tunica albuginea, the whitish fibrous sheath that encloses each testis.

whore a prostitute. The term has been used with this sense since the 12th century, but it is derived from the Latin word carus, meaning 'dear, beloved.'

widdle a euphemism meaning to urinate, used particularly by or to children.

widow Inheritance a practice found in many African societies: A man inherits all his dead father's wives except for his own mother. The object seems to be to carry on the family. In some parts of East Africa, the heir must go through the ritual of having intercourse with each of the wives in a single night on penalty of being required to renounce his father's property.

wife beating a common term referring to the battered-wife syndrome.

wife Inheritance a custom in which a man may be the principal heir of his mother's brother, including the mother's brother's wife or wives. The custom is found in many African societies; in some cases the inherited rights over the wife or wives may only be domestic, not sexual, though in other cases both sexual and domestic rights are inherited.

wife lending another term for sex hospitality.

willing an erection an aspect of the fear-of- failure process in secondary impotence in which a man who has failed to achieve an erection believes he should be able to produce an erection simply by will power,' even though he may have unintentionally obstructed the physiological requirements for an erection by an excessive intake of alcohol. The approach usually results in another failure, thereby reinforcing the problem.

willy a euphemism for penis, used particularly by or to children.

wimp an alternative term for cissy, or a male who lacks traditional masculine behavioural traits or who displays submissive or retiring characteristics.

winkle a euphemism for penis, used particularly by or to children.

wish fulfilment the realization of desires and goals—in psychoanalysis, one of the major mechanisms in dreams and fantasies; also the drive to find relief from tension produced by instinctual needs such as sex and hostility.

witches' milk a thin yellowish fluid resembling colostrum secreted by the breasts of newborn infants of both sexes. The secretion is normal, harmless, and transient.

withdrawal bleeding the discharge of blood from the uterus after a woman stops using a hormonal medication taken to evaluate the cause of her amenorrhoea symptoms. By taking progesterone for several days, then discontinuing the hormone, a discharge resembling a menstrual flow is a sign that the cause of the amenorrhoea is riot the result of a uterine disorder. The process is similar to the progesterone test for pregnancy.

withdrawal method a contraceptive method in which the male withdraws the penis from the vagina just before ejaculation. This technique is not reliable because the penis often releases semen containing sperm even before ejaculation, and because many men find it difficult to withdraw near the peak of sexual excitement. If possible, withdrawal should be delayed until the woman reaches a climax, otherwise it might interfere with her gratification.

witness a term referring to the origin of the term to testify,' because in ancient times it was customary for a man to place his hand on his testicles when taking an oath. Thus, the term, 'testify' is derived from 'testes,' and the testicles were 'witnesses' to the man's oath.

wolf an obsolescent slang term for a sexually aggressive male.

wolfflan duct a paired mesonephric tube that appears in the embryo and in the male evolves into the vas deference and a portion of the epididymis. In the female, the wolffian duct usually, but not always, degenerates and disappears.

woman an adult human female. The term comes from Old English wifeman, or 'female man;' nevertheless, woman has become the term preferred in the women's liberation movement, over other terms such as girl or lady (although the latter would seem to have more dignity, etymologically speaking—coming from Old English hlaefdige, 'loaf kneader, kneader of bread,' thus the indispensable provider of the family). But, then, usage has always been more important than literal sense. Willard R. Espy muses: 'The very word woman has become offensive in some circles, lady has come down to where woman was a hundred years ago, and in two thousand years, carus, Latin for 'dear.' has degenerated to whore. A courtesan was once a lady at court; a wench any young girl; tart, a term of endearment. Even housewife, that most respectable of appellations, becomes opprobrious when pronounced hussy.

womandrake a counterfeit version of man drake once offered in England. It actually was carved from the roots of a bryony vine and decorated with 'pubic hair' made from grass or wheat stalks.

womanizer a colloquial term for a man who habitually chases women.

woman-year a statistical term used in deter mining the comparative effectiveness of various kinds of birth-control methods. A woman-year represents 12 months in the life of a sexually active woman of an age between menarche and menopause, or who is at risk of becoming pregnant

womb a common synonym for uterus.

womb envy a form of envy experienced by male transsexuals who identify themselves so completely with the female sex that the they persistent desire to possess a womb.

womb fantasy the fantasy of returning the womb usually in response to the wish escape from the world and its pressures. According to Freud, this wish is usually expressed in symbolic form as a dream about living in a cave, being alone on an island, being confined to an empty room.

woman at risk women who are exposed the risk of pregnancy, such as low-income women, teenage girls, and others who for various reasons do not have access to contraceptive methods or services.

woman with penis the psychoanalytical concept that some children between the ages of 2 and 5 believe that all women once possessed a penis. Among girls this idea is a denial of reality stemming from the discovery of the anatomical differences between males and females. Among boys the discovery that girls lack a penis reinforces their anxiety about castration.

woodruff a small perennial herb that is used in the production of medicinal drugs. It has also been claimed over the centuries as a mild aphrodisiac; or, as one natural scientist noted in the 17th century, Woodruff is 'provocative to venery.'

working girl a euphemism for prostitute.

wrong door a slang term for anus, used in the context of anal sex.

wrongful birth the birth of an unwanted child, a situation that has been the basis of lawsuits against doctors, hospitals, clinics, and other health-care workers or facilities. The action may result from a failed vasectomy or tubal ligation leading to a pregnancy.

X

X chromosome the female sex chromosome. It is present in all ova and in half of all spermatozoa; the other half of the spermatozoa contain the Y, or male, sex chromosome. Female somatic (body) cells normally contain two X chromosomes, although one is inactivated.

X-linked abnormality any genetic disorder that is transmitted by a-gene on an X chromosome. X-linked abnormalities are as manifested in the male whose sex-chromosome counterpart, the Y chromosome, has no matching genes for those on the female sex chromosome. The male may express an X-linked abnormality even though it is carried as a recessive gene.

X deletion a loss or deletion of part of the X chromosome of a female karyotype. It is not unusual for a portion of a chromosome to be lost during the cell divisions of meiosis or mitosis. The event often results in an offspring being born with an abnormality if the lost portion is not required for survival of the embryo. Authorities estimate that 75 per cent of all such chromosomal defects involve the sex chromosomes, resulting in such abnormalities as Turner's syndrome effects.

XXXXX syndrome a rare condition marked by the presence of three extra X chromosomes in a superfemale. The woman is generally normal in female physical characteristics, and fertile, but may exhibit some degree of mental retardation, ocular disorders, or limb abnormalities.

XXXXY syndrome one of the genetic expressions of Klinefelter's syndrome, usually characterized by a tall male with long legs but with poorly developed male genitalia, a deficiency of normal male secondary sexual characteristics, an absence of fertility, and in some cases mental retardation. Such individuals often are discovered after adulthood when they undergo medical tests to determine the reason for their infertility.

XXXY syndrome a variation of the Klinefelter syndrome in which the male possesses three X chromosomes, or a total of 48 chromosomes. The features of the Klinefelter individual who is trisomic for the X chromosome are similar to those of the 49,XXXXY male.

XXY syndrome a condition that is the most common form of Klinefelter's syndrome. With a chromosome count of 47, as compared with the normal total of 46, the individual usually possesses enough Y chromosome influence to acquire the basic male features although disomic for the X chromosome. The additional -X chromosome is generally not detected or expressed until after puberty. The XXY complement occurs about once in every 500 male births.

XXYY syndrome a male who is disomic for both the X and Y chromosomes. He may have some of the features found in Klinefelter's syndrome, particularly testicular dysgenesis and sterility.

Y

yang and yin according to ancient Chinese doctrine, two fundamental forces that pervade the universe and control human life. They represent such opposites as masculine-feminine, active-passive, moon-sun, and earth-heaven. Sexually speaking, the yang force of Heaven is dominant in men and determines the outer shape of the male sex organ, and the yin force of Earth is dominant in women and determines the inward shape of the female sex organ. These two forces complement each other during sexual contact, and a balanced, cosmic harmony is believed to result.

yantra in the Hindu tradition, a mystic six pointed diagram composed of two superim- posed triangles that symbolize the harmonious balance between the five senses (touch, sound, sight, taste and smell), the mind, and the male and female functions. The diagram is used as a meditation device in creating a harmony of emotions, as an aid in performing rituals, and as a protective talisman.

Yapese inhabitants of a large island in the Carolines whose diet depends on fishing. The society is mainly monogamous, though polygyny is permitted. Their customs and beliefs include insistence that a man is unnecessary for procreation; an intercourse position in which a man is seated and the woman squats on top facing him and urinates as she reaches orgasm; blackening of the teeth as a form of beautification; the view that incest is something that animals do, not human beings, and that a woman who has committed incest cannot bear children; erotic festivals involving sexual licence and public outdoor copulation; the practice of coitus interruptus, possibly for birth control; a taboo against intercourse during menstruation; a unique taboo against bathing in the ocean after intercourse.

yarrow a common herb that grows it, much of the world between the tropics and the Arctic Circles. It is also known by its common name of staunch-wound, which reveals its links to medieval witchcraft. Yarrow was traditionally used at weddings to ensure 7 years of true love. Young women in Europe and America used to believe that if tickling their nostrils with yarrow caused a nosebleed it meant their lovers were faithful.

Y chromosome the male sex chromosome, which is present in half of all spermatozoa while none is found in a female gamete or a normal female body cell The main function of the Y chromosome is believed to be the synthesis of molecules that lead to production of male sex hormones, which in turn result in the physical characteristics of the male sex. All males require an X chromosome in addition to the Y chromosome.

yellow body the corpus luteum of the ovary.

Y-linked pertaining to the genes or traits carried by the male sex chromosome. Certain characteristics, such as hair on the external ear, are Y-linked and are expressed only in males.

yohimbine an alkaloid obtained from the bark of the yohimbe tree (Pausinystalia yohimba), which grows in west central Africa. It is used as an alleged aphrodisiac. Yohimbine has been discovered to be identical with quebrachine, obtained from white quebracho bark. The name is western African in origin.

yolk sac an embryonic structure formed by cells that extend into the cavity of the blastocyst. In lower animals, the yolk sac contains nutrients that sustain life and growth of the embryo. In humans, the yolk sac is a rudimentary bit of tissue that provides little or no nourishment to the beginning embryo which obtains its nutrients by osmosis from the blood lakes in the walls of the uterus.

yolk stalk a threadlike structure that con- nects the embryo to the yolk sac.

yonl the Hindu name for the female sex organ (vagina), which is worshipped in Tantric rites throughout India. The yoni is depicted in sculpture placed at Hindu shrines, and its likeness is frequently worn as an amulet.

Z

Z chromosome a male sex chromosome of some birds, fishes, and insects with male disomic sex chromosomes. In such species it is the male that possesses the duplicate (ZZ) sex chromosomes while the female sex characteristics are determined by a combination of one W and one Z sex chromosome.

Zina a Muslim category for all forbidden sex acts, including bestiality, prostitution, anal sex, and lesbianism. The penalty for Zina violations is death.

zinc deficiency a condition resulting from a lack of zinc in the diet. Effects include a loss of taste and smell sensitivity, fatigue, and delayed sexual maturity. There also is evidence that zinc contributes to normal sexuality. Because oysters and other seafood can be a good source of zinc, it has been suggested that its presence may be the basis for claims that seafoods may have aphrodisiac qualities.

zip Injury of the penis a painful injury caused by catching the excess skin of the penis in the zip of a trouser fly. The recommended treatment is to sedate the victim, then deaden the sensitivity of the penis with a generous amount of Nupercainal ointment. If necessary, the zip is cut away from the trousers to manipulate it away from the skin without causing added injury.

zipper ring an intrauterine contraceptive device made of coils of nylon thread. Its claimed advantage is that it can be inserted without prior mechanical dilation of the cervix.

zona fasciculata a layer of the adrenal gland cortex in which androgenic sex hormones are produced.

zone pellucida a thick, transparent, protective membrane that is secreted round the ovum during its maturation in an ovary. The membrane is produced by the cytoplasm of the ovum and remains with the ovum until after fertilization.

zooerasty sexual excitement or gratification through contact with an animal.

zoolagnia sexual pleasure from contacts with animals.

zoophilla a psychosexual disorder in which farm animals or household pets are persistently preferred or exclusively used to achieve sexual excitement.

zoosadist a person who derives sexual pleasure from injuring animals.

Zovirax a brand name for the drug acyclovir approved by the US Food and Drug Administration in 1985 as a medication for the treatment of genital herpes.

Zulu a South African society in which polygyny is (or was) the general rule, preferably the sororal type. Among their customs is (or was) the-removal of all hair in the pubic and armpit regions by both men and women; rituals in which unmarried women dance 4 bare-breasted and wearing nothing but beads, to show that their bodies are not flabby, which would be an indication of sexual immorality; punishment for adultery by flogging the offenders with thorny branches, and in some cases thrusting cacti into the women's vagina; a taboo against daylight intercourse—otherwise people would 'behave like dogs'; and various other taboos such as avoidance of sex during a storm, after a bad dream, or after the husband has killed a python, crocodile, or hyena.

zygote the fertilized ovum, containing both sets of chromosomes from the male and female gametes, before it begins to divide.